Testbank to Accompany

Pharmacology

Drug Therapy and Nursing Considerations

Julia Robinson, RN, MS, FNP
Professor
Department of Nursing
California State University, Bakersfield
Bakersfield , CA

Barbara Mouser, MSN, CRRN
Lecturer
Department Of Nursing
California State University, Bakersfield
Bakersfield, CA

Fourth Edition

J.B. Lippincott Company
Philadelphia

D1211694

Sponsoring Editor: Margaret Belcher
Editorial Assistant: Emily Cotlier
Ancillary Coordinator: Doris S. Wray
Compositor: DTP Inc.
Printer/Binder: Courier-Kendalville

ISBN 0-397-55201-7

6 5 4 3 2 1

Any procedure or practice described in this book should be applied by the healthcare practitioner under appropriate supervision in accordance with professional standards of care used with regard to the unique circumstances that apply in each practice situation. Care has been taken to confirm the accuracy of information presented and to describe generally accepted practices. However, the authors, editors, and publisher cannot accept any responsibility for errors or omissions or for any consequences from application of the information in this book and make not warranty express or implied with respect to the contents of the book.

Every effort has been made to ensure drug selections and dosages are in accordance with current recommendations and practice. Because of ongoing research, changes in government regulations, and the constant flow of information on drug therapy, reactions, and interactions, the reader is cautioned to check the package insert for each drug for indications, dosages, warnings, and precautions, particularly if the drug is new or infrequently used.

Contents

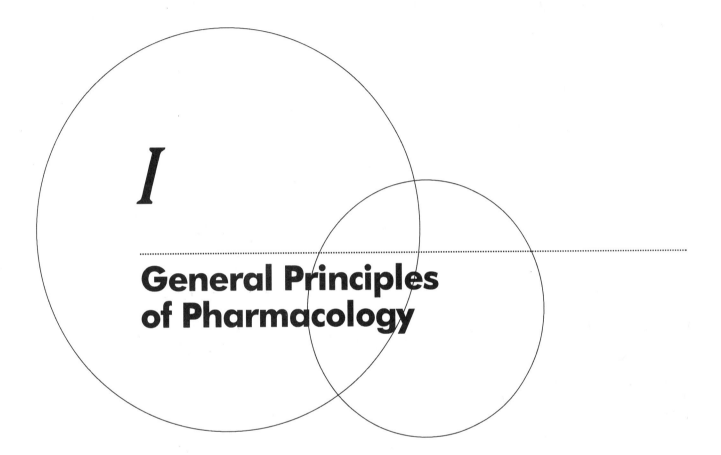

I

General Principles of Pharmacology

1
The Nurse's Role in the Management of Drug Therapy

1. Nursing management of patients for whom drug therapy is prescribed includes a careful medication history including investigation of the use of OTC drugs because these drugs:

   a. are often as effective as the prescribed drug therapy.

   *b. might be being used to mask side-effects of prescribed drugs.

   c. are often ineffective in producing the intended effect.

   d. will all need to be discontinued promptly for safety reasons.

   Reference: p. 4

2. Nursing interventions for management of patients on prescribed drug therapy includes obtaining a history of alcohol intake for all of the following purposes *except*:

   a. drug effects may be additive in the presence of alcohol.

   b. drug effects may be decreased by concurrent alcohol use.

   *c. all alcohol consumption will need to be discontinued.

   d. a possible need for cautious use of drugs may be uncovered.

   Reference: p. 4

3. Nursing assessment of the patient for whom drugs are prescribed includes determining whether or not the individual of reproductive age is pregnant in order to determine a benefit-to-risk ratio.
   Drugs that have shown positive evidence of adverse risk to the human fetus are categorized in the Food and Drug Administration (FDA) Pregnancy Category:

   a. C.

   *b. D.

   c. X.

   d. NR.

   Reference: p. 5

4. Taking a medication history from the patient for whom a drug is being prescribed includes carefully reviewing possible contraindication to its use based on known hypersensitivity to a particular drug or the drugs within a drug category. Allergic reactions that include skin eruptions, painful joints, and drug fever are categorized as:

   a. Type I.

   b. Type II.

   *c. Type III.

   d. Type IV.

   Reference: p. 6

5. Mary O'Neal, a 55 year old patient with insulin dependent diabetes and hypertension, is admitted for an emergency cholecystectomy. The patient says to the nurse, "I am allergic to penicillin." Which question by the nurse is likely elicit the most information for assessment purposes?

   *a. "Describe the type of reaction that occurs."

   b. "Did this occur after the first dose or after several?"

   c. "Do you develop a headache when the allergy occurs?"

   d. "Are you allergic to other substances as animal dander ?"

   Reference: p. 6

6. The nursing diagnosis that most likely applies to 55 year old mechanic newly diagnosed with non-insulin dependent diabetes mellitus and who is eager to get started on his oral hypoglycemic agent "in order to feel better" is:

   a. High risk for noncompliance with drug therapy related to anxiety secondary to complexity of therapeutic regimen.

   *b. Knowledge deficit regarding drug therapy related to unfamiliarity with purposes, side effects, etc. of drug.

c. Potential complication: Ketoacidosis related to knowledge deficit.

d. High risk for altered health maintenance related to insufficient knowledge to manage condition.

Reference: p. 8

7. When taking a medication history on the patient, which of the following questions would most effectively elicit information relative to their level of compliance?

a. "What are the names, and dosages of the drugs you take?"

*b. "Tell me about your daily routine in taking medications."

c. "Are you experiencing any side-effects from your drugs?"

d. "Does your family remind you to take your medications?"

Reference: p. 9

8. A statement by a patient is indicative that s/he is at increased risk for noncompliance to drug therapy is:

a. "I take my own blood pressure and record the readings."

b. "I forget to take my pill at the same time every day."

*c. "My arthritis makes it difficult to open containers."

d. "Grandfather had high blood pressure and lived to be 90!"

Reference: p. 10

9. Nursing intervention includes health teaching that promotes patient compliance to the prescribed medication regimen. An indication that a patient with newly diagnosed essential hypertension is ready to learn about their drug therapy is the individual:

a. is able to cite the names and dosages of the drugs prescribed.

b. is able to cite the needs and benefits of the medication.

*c. accepts the diagnosis and understands its adverse effects.

d. says "my spouse will remind me to take of my drugs."

Reference: p. 10

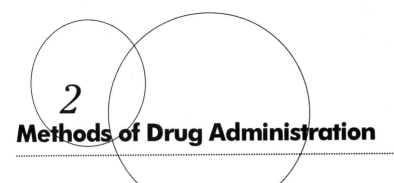

2
Methods of Drug Administration

1. Dr. Smith has ordered Septra 160 mg q 12 h po for Mrs. Jones' UTI. Before giving the first dose of this medication to her, it is *most* important for the nurse to determine:

   a. how rapidly the medication is absorbed.

   b. the urgency of the patient's need for the medication.

   c. the appropriateness of the ordered route.

   *d. the presence of allergies.

   Reference: p. 12

2. In general, when educating the patient in taking his medication, the best instruction is to:

   a. take the medication until a "steady state" of blood medication level has been reached, and then discontinue the drug.

   *b. take the medication until the prescription is finished.

   c. take medications with meals to enhance absorption.

   d. take medications until symptoms have been eradicated.

   Reference: p.12

3. Care must be taken in the administration of drugs through the mucous membranes because:

   *a. many drugs exert significant systemic action after application to the mucous membranes.

   b. medications are absorbed more slowly through the mucous membranes than through the skin.

   c. many drugs applied to the mucous membranes exert only local effects.

   d. generalized adverse reactions are not a concern with drugs that are applied to the mucous membranes.

   Reference: p. 13

4. A problem encountered with administration of drugs rectally is that:

   a. the rectal route cannot be used for an uncooperative patient.

   b. the rectal mucosa is extremely sensitive and very few medications are given in this manner.

   *c. drug absorption from the rectal route is unpredictable.

   d. it is necessary to give a soapsuds enema before rectal administration of any medication.

   Reference: p. 13

5. Sublingual nitroglycerine has been ordered for your patient. She is having trouble taking the medication because her mouth is so dry. You instruct her:

   a. to place the tablet under her tongue, then as it dissolves, to drink a glass of water.

   *b. to rinse the mouth with water, then place the tablet beneath the tongue.

   c. to place the tablet in the cheek, next to the molars, where the moistening effect of saliva is greater.

   d. to chew the tablet in order to moisten it, then hold in the mouth until it absorbs.

   Reference: p. 14

7. When instilling ear drops, it is important to remember to:

   a. use a cool solution.

   b. position the patient with the affected ear down for several minutes after instilling drops.

   c. pull the pinna up and back if the patient is a child is under three years old.

   *d. pull the pinna down and back if the patient is a child under three years old.

   Reference: p. 15

8. Your patient is taking anti-glaucoma eye drops for the first time. You know that it is important to instruct the her to:

   a. use sterile technique in instilling the drops, as the packaging is sterile.

   *b. use the drops as ordered to prevent deterioration of vision.

    c. remember that the drops will dilate the pupil and the use of dark glasses is advisable.

    d. to place the drops directly on the cornea to enhance the effects of the medication.

Reference: p. 14

9. The largest fluid dose that can be given safely intramuscularly is:

    a. 2 ml

    b. 3 ml

    c. 4 ml

*d. 5 ml

Reference: p. 17

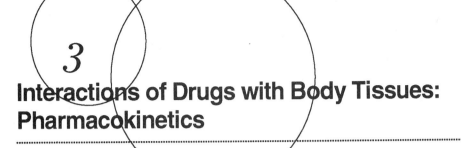

3
Interactions of Drugs with Body Tissues: Pharmacokinetics

1. Henry Clayton develops frequent premature ventricular contractions secondary to an acute myocardial infarction. The primary purpose for his physician prescribing lidocaine by IV bolus is:

    a. to decrease hepatic first-pass metabolism.

    *b. to achieve therapeutic levels quickly.

    c. to decrease the half-life of the drug.

    d. to maintain the drug in an ionized state.

    Reference: p. 22

2. Rose Mancasola is receiving enteric coated aspirin for treatment of her degenerative osteoarthritis. Enteric coatings on drugs:

    a. augment lipid solubility and absorption.

    b. diminish permeability of the GI mucosal epithelium.

    *c. resist breakdown and absorption in the stomach.

    d. increase hepatic "first pass" effects.

    Reference: p. 22

3. The body organ from which the excretion of drugs and their metabolites primarily occurs is the:

    *a. kidneys.

    b. intestines.

    c. skin.

    d. lungs.

    Reference: p. 24

4. Sue Bates has severe pancreatitis which caused in a severe curtailment of her food intake and resulting in an albumin level of 2.3 g/dl (normal: 3.8-5.0 g/dl). Because she is taking several drugs, hypoalbuminemia is of concern because there may be:

    a. delay in the rate of absorption from IM and SC sites.

    *b. insufficient binding sites for drug transportation.

    c. a decreased therapeutic effect from excess free drug.

    d. altered lipid solubility at the cell membrane.

    Reference: p. 23

5. An important property of an antibiotic used to treat meningitis would be:

    *a. lipid solubility and ability to cross the blood-brain barrier.

    b. high ionization and maximal protein binding in the plasma.

    c. lipid solubility and slow release from adipose tissue.

    d. a long half-life and rapid ionization at plasma pH.

    Reference: p. 23

6. Jesse Hayes, a 69 year old patient with a diagnosis of liver and chronic obstructive pulmonary disease is seen in the emergency room because of exacerbation of his COPD secondary to pneumonia. The nurse should observe Mr. Hayes for possible toxic drug effects primarily because of:

    a. decreased cardiac output.

    b prolonged gastric emptying.

    c. reduction in lung capacity.

    *d. altered liver function.

    Reference: p. 24

7. The reason for administering penicillin and probenecid together is to increase the therapeutic effectiveness of penicillin by:

    a. decreasing hepatic first-pass metabolism.

    *b. inhibiting tubular secretion.

    c. displacing protein binding sites.

    d. ionizing it in the tubular fluid.

    Reference: p. 24

8. Carla McCarthy is breast-feeding her newborn infant. Health teaching should include advising her to do all of the following *except:*

    a. to avoid taking over-the-counter drugs.

    b. to take only drugs prescribed by a healthcare provider

    c. to inform healthcare providers that she is breast feeding.

   *d. to supplement breast feeding just in case she becomes ill.

Reference: p. 25

9. Assuming a patient is receiving the correct dosage of morphine for pain that is difficult to control, a fairly constant blood level (*steady state*) of the drug will be achieved after the drug has been given:

    a. every 6 hours for 2 doses.

    b. every 4 hours for 3 doses.

    c. every 4 hours for 4 doses.

   *d. every 4 hours for 5 doses.

Reference: p. 25

4
Basic Sites and Mechanisms of Drug Actions: Pharmacodynamics

1. Agents that produce their effects by altering the rate of normal organ functions (pharmacodynamic effect) include all of the following except:
   *a. antibiotics
   b. diuretics
   c. antiarrhythmics
   d. antihypertensive
   Reference: p. 26

2. The "therapeutic index" for a given drug is:
   a. a way of adjusting dosage to body weight.
   b. a measure of the rate of drug accumulation.
   *c. a measure of its margin of safety
   d. a way to evaluate drug efficacy.
   Reference: p. 26

3. Luke Witham, a 70 year old male with a provisional diagnosis of renal calculi, is scheduled for an intravenous urogram. He tells the nurse, "I guess the doctor forgot that I had a severe reaction to the dye the last time this was done." The nurse implements measures to delay the test until the physician is consulted based on the rationale that:
   *a. there is a possibility that the patient is allergic to the drug.
   b. it is likely the patient doesn't think the test is necessary. c. a patient's expectations will result in a poor outcome.
   d. patients have the best knowledge of their response to a drug.
   Reference: p. 27

4. A patient who has developed tolerance to a drug exhibits:

   a. impaired response to a drug dose that is normally effective.
   b. a genetically determined unexpected response to a drug.
   * c. a decreased physiological response to repeated doses.
   d. a progressively increasing response to repeated doses.
   Reference: p. 27

5. Aden Jones receives naloxone (Narcan) to reverse the respiratory depression associated with postoperative opiate use for pain. This is an example of modifying the effects of one drug by another through the process of:
   a. inactivation of a drug by chemical complexing.
   b. one drug countering the biologic effects of another.
   c. reduced/blocked effects of one drug by another.
   *d. competition for the same receptor sites
   Reference: p. 28

6. Jon Byron, a 77 year old patient with congestive heart failure and renal dysfunction who is receiving digoxin 0.125 mg daily, develops digitalis toxicity. When a drug is excreted more slowly than it is absorbed the result is:
   a. tolerance.
   *b. cumulation
   c. idiosyncrasy
   d. resistence
   Reference: p. 28

5
Pharmacological Basis of Adverse Drug Effects

1. Overdosage with a therapeutic agent will elicit an excessive reaction to the *primary* effect of the drug. An example of this is:

   a. Agranulocytosis due to Chloramphenicol

   b. GI ulceration created by Aspirin

   c. Anaphylaxis caused by Penicillin

   *d. Excessive electrolyte depletion with Lasix.

   Reference: p. 30

2. Mrs Jones is beginning a regime of Aspirin gr. XV tid for her worsening osteoarthritis. While you are formulating her health history, you are keeping in mind that this is a very commonly used drug. You know that in view of the frequency of use in general:

   *a. A complete health history is important to ensure giving the aspirin safely.

   b. Some components of the health history can be omitted because aspirin is such a frequently used drug.

   c. The history needs to include complete blood counts and liver panels.

   d. The health history is not as important as follow-up monitoring to detect untoward effects.

   Reference: p. 32

3. The role of the liver in the metabolism of many drugs is:

   a. breakdown of the drug into its major components.

   b. synthesis of the drug into the bloodstream.

   *c. inactivation of the drug at the hepatic level.

   d. absorption of the drug at the cellular level.

   Reference: p. 32

4. The presence of renal disease can cause many ADRs (adverse drug reactions) to be produced by those drugs that are eliminated largely through the renal system. These reactions are caused by:

   *a. an increase in the unbound (free) levels of the drug.

   b. an increase in plasma protein levels.

   c. an alteration in the chemical components of the drug.

   d. an alteration in the peak-trough cycle.

   Reference: p. 32

5. The most commonly observed drug induced manifestation of hepatotoxicity is:

   a. ascites

   *b. jaundice

   c. edema

   d. photosensitivity

   Reference: p. 33

6. Extrapyramidial reactions are frequently associated with the use of:

   a. aminoglycoside antibiotics

   b. certain diuretics

   c. sedatives

   *d. antipsychotic drugs

   Reference: p. 33

7. The most common drug-induced blood dyscrasia is:

   a. aplastic anemia.

   b. thrombocytopenia.

   *c. agranulocytosis.

   d. hemolytic anemia.

   Reference: p. 33

9. Ototoxicity is observed most commonly as an adverse reaction to these drugs:

   *a. aminoglycoside antibiotics and some diuretics.

   b. some cephalosporins and antipsychotics.

   c. calcium-channel blockers and benzo-diazepines.

   d. corticosteroids and some narcotics.

   Reference: p. 33

10. The most common manifestation of ocular toxicity is:

   a. myopia.

*b. blurred vision.

   c. scotomata.

   d. amblyopia.

Reference: p. 33

6
Drug Interactions

1. Physiological factors that can greatly influence the frequency of drug interactions include all of the following *except*:
   a. genetic abnormalities.
   b. weight.
   c. sex.
   *d. pollutant exposure.
   Reference: p. 35

2. Precipitation of amphotericin when it is mixed with normal saline instead of 5% dextrose is an example of:
   a. chemical incompatibility.
   *b. physical incompatibility.
   c. competitive antagonism.
   d. enzyme induction.
   Reference: p. 36

3. A synergistic pharmacodynamic drug interaction results from:
   a. inhibition of active transport mechanisms by two drugs that compete for these processes.
   b. cancelling the effects of one drug by the use of a second one that blocks the receptor site of the first one.
   *c. the enhancement of the effects of one drug by another that has similar actions.
   d. two drugs with opposing actions which reduces or abolishes the effects of each.
   Reference: p. 36

4. The full effects of a sustained-release dosage form of a drug may be markedly altered by the concurrent use of drugs that:
   a. increase bile flow.
   b. decrease GI motility.
   *c. increase GI motility.
   d. decrease gastric pH.
   Reference: p. 37

5. A number of factors alter gastrointestinal drug absorption. The process by which fat-soluble drugs, such as vitamins A, D, and K, are taken up by mineral oil thereby decreasing their absorption is termed:
   a. chemical binding.
   *b. sequestration.
   c. protein binding.
   d. enzyme inhibition.
   Reference: p. 37

6. Prior to suturing a deep laceration on a patient, the physician injects a lidocaine combined with epinephrine around the wound. This is an example of combining two drugs:
   *a. to restrict spread into the systemic circulation by vasoconstriction.
   b. to modify the toxic effects of one drug by antagonizing these by another one.
   c. to slow absorption by forming an insoluble complex by chemical binding.
   d. to produce an additive effect and increase the degree of local anesthesia.
   Reference: p. 38

7. An example of *enzyme induction* involving biotransformation and thereby producing a drug interaction is:
   a. elevation of biogenic enzymes with the use of MAO inhibitors.
   *b. rapid metabolism of coumarin in the presence of barbiturates.
   c. blockage of degradation of choline esters by neostigmine.
   d. prolonged reduction in enzyme activity 2 weeks after the an MAO inhibitor is discontinued.
   Reference: p. 38

7
Therapeutic Drug Monitoring

1. Bioavailability of a drug at any given dose is maximized by administering it:

   a. sublingual.

   b. oral.

   *c. intravenous.

   d. intramuscular.

   Reference: p. 40

2. Arthur Lum is seen in the emergency room for a moderately severe bronchitis. The physician prescribes non-enteric coated erythromycin 250 mg P.O. every 6 hours. To maximize its absorption the nurse should instruct Mr. Lum to take the drug:

   a. with food during meals and a snack at bedtime.

   *b. with water 2 hours after meals and at bedtime.

   c. a glass of milk 1 hour before meals and at bedtime.

   d. an antacid 2 hours after meals and at bedtime.

   Reference: p. 43

3. The half-life of digoxin, the medication Sue Jerold's physician has prescribed to treat her congestive heart failure, is approximately 36 hours. The "half-life" of a drug means the time required for the drug:

   a. to be cleared by the kidneys.

   b. to produce a therapeutic response.

   c. to reach its therapeutic potential.

   *d. serum level to be reduced by one-half.

   Reference: p. 42

4. Simone McGlynn is receiving digoxin for congestive heart failure. Following 3-4 days of therapy, her physician orders a drug serum level for the purpose of determining:

   a. a possible need for a loading dose.

   b. the ideal dose for body weight.

   *c. the desirable therapeutic levels.

   d. the half-life of the drug.

   Reference: p. 42

5. A nurse administering a drug with a half life of 6 hours knows that the steady state serum level of the drug will be reached when the patient has received it:

   a. every 4 hours for 20 hours.

   b. every 4 hours for 32 hours.

   c. every 6 hours for 24 hours.

   *d. every 6 hours for 30 hours.

   Reference: p. 42

6. The physician orders a "trough level" for gentamicin after a patient has received 3 intravenous doses at 8 hour intervals over a 24 hour period. To determine this, blood should be obtained:

   a. immediately after the next dose.

   b. two hours after the next dose.

   c. four hours after the next dose.

   *d. prior to giving the next dose,

   Reference: p. 42

7. A major factor known to contribute to differences among patients in the volume of distribution of drugs in the body is:

   a. the speed and/or amount of drug absorbed.

   b. differences in the rate of drug metabolism.

   *c. the changes in the protein binding of drugs.

   d. the elimination half-life of the drugs.

   Reference: p. 43

8. The benefits of therapeutic drug monitoring for the patient include all of the following *except*:

   a. with rapid drug therapy, dosing rate is assessed quickly.

   b. with an added drug, change in one drug level is assessed.

   c. determines optimal therapy with minimum/no toxicity.

 *d. reassurance that the physician is doing his best.

   Reference: p. 44

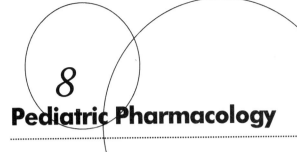

8
Pediatric Pharmacology

1. The most critical period in the child's growth stages as far as drug handling is:

   *a. The neonatal period (0-1 months)

   b. Infancy (2-12 months)

   c. Toddler (13 months-36 months)

   d. Preschool (3 years to 5 years)

   Reference: p. 46

2. The well-informed nurse's knows that the response to medication in the infant and young child is influenced by factors that include the following concept:

   a. Infants under 6 months of age absorb orally administered drugs rapidly.

   b. All nutrients and vitamins are well absorbed by young infants.

   *c. The absorption of topically applied drugs is enhanced in children as compared to adults.

   d. Drugs are well absorbed from intramuscular sites in infants.

   Reference: p. 46

3. Three week old Todd has developed a high fever and upper respiratory distress. He is to be hospitalized for antibiotic therapy to treat the infection and for the treatment of dehydration. The *best* route for the administration of the antibiotic under these circumstances is:

   a. in the gluteus maximus because of the increased blood supply to the muscles.

   b. p.o. because of the rapid absorption from this route.

   *c. I.V. in 500 ml of fluid for uniform absorption.

   d. in the vastus lateralis muscle of the thigh because of the better blood supply.

   Reference: p. 49

4. Hepatic drug metabolism is lower in the early neonatal period allowing larger unbound quantities of a drug to circulate. In order to achieve safe dosing, the nurse will administer:

   a. more frequent doses in smaller amounts to minimize fluctuating blood levels.

   b. combinations of drugs to avoid enzymatic breakdown of the medications.

   *c. smaller doses of the drug to avoid toxic accumulation.

   d. larger doses of the drug as unmetabolized medication is not utilized by the body.

   Reference: p. 47

5. Drug dosage for the young child is most *accurately* calculated based upon:

   a. the age of the child.

   b. the size of the child.

   c. the weight of the child.

   *d. the surface area of the child.

   Reference: p. 48

6. Your young (2 1/2 year old patient is not happy about taking her liquid Ampicillin. In order to insure that she gets the medication she needs, you employ the following strategy:

   a. You mix the Ampicillin in her orange juice so that she won't realize that she is taking medicine.

   *b. You ask if she would like the Ampicillin in a grape flavored juice or strawberry flavor.

   c. You promise her a candy treat if she takes her medication.

   d. You firmly insist that the child swallow the medication, spooning it into her mouth if necessary.

   Reference: p. 49

9
Geriatric Pharmacology

1. In eliciting a drug history from a Marie Rogers, a 72 year old patient, she reports taking medications from each of the following categories. When taken concurrently with other drug, those likely to affect the amount of drug entering the blood stream are:

   a. diuretics.

   b. digestants.

   *c. laxatives.

   d. analgesics.

   Reference: p. 51

2. In relation to altered drug responses in the elderly, the variable most likely to in be influenced by changes in the levels of plasma proteins (albumin) is:

   a. absorption.

   b. metabolism.

   *c. distribution.

   d. elimination.

   Reference: p. 51

3. The major age-related change that increases the elimination half-life of most drugs in the elderly is:

   a. decreased intestinal peristalsis.

   b. increased tubular secretion.

   *c. decreased liver enzyme activity.

   d. decreased blood albumin.

   Reference: p. 51

4. An age-related change responsible for the powerful effects of the benzodiazepines that occurs in the elderly patient is:

   *a. altered tissue sensitivity.

   b. diminished tubular reabsorption.

   c. decreased blood albumin.

   d. chronic disease states.

   Reference: p. 52

5. A nurse in an outpatient clinic for the elderly assesses Rapher Regor, a 68 year old man taking an antihypertensive, a diuretic, a NSAID, and an antidepressant, for possible causes of recent mental changes (short term memory loss and mental confusion). A primary consideration should be:

   *a. developing drug toxicity.

   b. worsening of depression.

   c. excessively low blood pressure.

   d. dehydration due to diuresis.

   Reference: p. 52

6. Diminished endogenous hormones in the elderly require cautious initiation/use of the therapeutic use of hormones. In the elderly, the use of glucocorticoids are known to be associated with all of the following effects *except:*

   a. greater susceptibility to infection.

   b. diminished response to antidiabetic agents.

   c. the development of osteoporosis.

   *d. rapid development of cataracts.

   Reference: p. 52

7. Nellie Frank, who is 85 years old and lives independently in her own apartment near her daughter's residence, takes several drugs. The patient's statement that is most indicative of a possible problem with compliance to the prescribed regimen is:

   a. "My doctor explained my condition and the need for drugs."

   b. "I keep a record of what I am supposed to take when."

   c. "I keep my drugs near where I make coffee in the morning."

   *d. "My vision is blurred and I need to have my eyes checked."

   Reference: p.52

10
Legal Aspects of Drug Therapy

1. In the United States official drugs that conform to given standards for strength, quality, purity, packaging safety, and labeling are listed in the:
   a. *Physicians' Desk Reference*
   *b. *United States Pharmacopoeia and National Formulary*
   c. *Drugs Facts and Comparisons*
   d. *American Hospital Formulary Service*

   Reference: p. 55

2. "Legend drugs" are those that are:
   a. over-the-counter drugs sold without a prescription in drug stores.
   b. substances as vitamins, nutrients that are sold in health food stores.
   c. folk remedies used in traditional medicine by various cultures.
   *d. drugs obtained by prescription from a qualified healthcare provider.

   Reference: p. 55

3. Dispensing of certain substances by pharmacists and pharmacist interns is provided for by the Controlled Substances Act of 1970 in the drug classification category of:
   a. Schedule II.
   b. Schedule III.
   c. Schedule IV.
   *d. Schedule V.

   Reference: p. 57

4. Policies that directly affect nursing responsibilities related to the administration of controlled drugs within healthcare institutions include of all of the following *except:*
   *a. verifying correctness of the dose of Schedule II drugs with another qualified nurse.
   b. making sure that controlled drugs are kept in a locked cabinet with limited access.

   c. observing patients' responses to drugs and reporting significant changes to the physician.
   d. documenting the patient's response to the drug each time it is administered.

   Reference: p. 58

5. Drugs available by prescription are grouped into one of four categories. Those having mood-altering effects that are likely to become habit forming but excluding most anxiolytics are classified as:
   a. schedule F.
   *b. schedule G.
   c. narcotic drugs.
   d. schedule H.
   Reference: p. 58

6. Drugs that may be dispensed only on written prescription and that cannot be refilled are those belonging to the category of:
   a. schedule F.
   b. schedule G.
   *c. narcotic drugs.
   d. schedule H.
   Reference: p. 58

7. A hospice nurse suspects that a Schedule II opiate based analgesic prescribed for a terminally ill patient is being taken by a member of the patient's family. Which of the following would be the most appropriate initial action by the nurse?
   a. Reveal this suspicion directly to the family member in question.
   *b. Phone the pharmacist and ask about the frequency of refills of the drug.
   c. Phone the patient's physician and ask if she/he can identify the suspect.
   d. Report the matter to the a narcotics regulatory agency within 24 hours.

   Reference: p. 59

8. Depending upon state statute, people empowered to write prescriptions besides physicians may include all of the following *except*:

    *a. chiropractors.

    b. veterinarians.

    c. nurse practitioners.

    d. dentists.

    Reference: p. 59

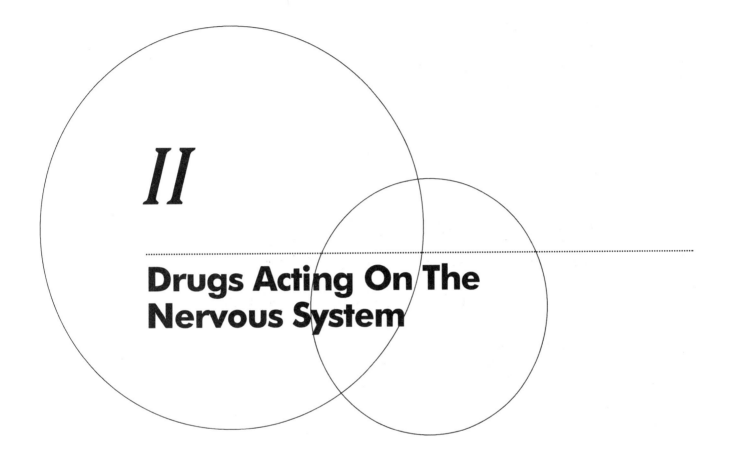

II

Drugs Acting On The Nervous System

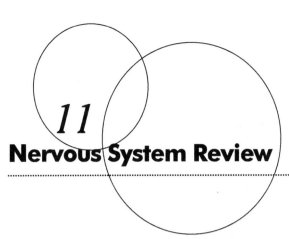

11
Nervous System Review

1. The cholinergic or parasympathetic nervous system transmits messages through:
   *a. The action of acetylcholine.
   b. The action of norepinephrine.
   c. The action of polypeptides.
   d. The action of serotonin.
   Reference: p. 63

2. The sympathetic, or adrenergic nervous system transmits messages through the action of:
   a. acetylcholine.
   *b. norepinephrine.
   c. polypeptides.
   d. serotonin.
   Reference: p. 63

3. The production of most neurotransmitters is inhibited by:
   a. the arrival of a nerve action potential.
   b. depolarization of the presynaptic membrane.
   c. influx of calcium ions into the nerve endings.
   *d. increase in the level of the neurotransmitter.
   Reference: p. 66

4. The principal means of the breakdown of the neurotransmitter acetylcholine is accomplished by:
   a. diffusion of the neurotransmitter away from the synaptic area.
   b. enzymatic breakdown of the neurotransmitter by monoamine oxidase.
   c. uptake of the transmitter into smooth muscle cells.
   *d. enzymatic breakdown of the transmitter by acetylcholinesterase.
   Reference: p. 66

5. Norepinephrine is an Alpa 1 activator. Its expected action would be:
   a. Retention of liposomes within the fat cells.
   b. Relaxation of smooth muscle cells

   *c. Release of glycogen from the liver.
   d. Release of insulin from the pancreas.
   Reference: p. 65

6. The principal means of the breakdown of the neurotransmitter norepinephrine is accomplished by:
   a. the uptake of the transmitter into the glial cells.
   b. enzymatic breakdown of the neurotransmitter by MAO and COMT.
   *c. uptake of the neurotransmitter into the presynaptic nerve endings.
   d. activation of presynaptic alpha 2 receptors.

   Reference: p. 65

7. Cholinergic receptors are identified as:
   a. Alpha 1 and Alpha 2 receptors.
   *b. Muscarinic and Nicotinic receptors.
   c. Beta 1 and Beta 2 receptors.
   d. Dopamine receptors.

   Reference: p. 66

8. Dopamine receptors are located in the:
   *a. kidney.
   b. liver.
   c. pancreas.
   d. eye.

   Reference: p. 66

9. M receptor sites are found in the:
   a. kidney.
   b. skeletal muscle.
   *c. smooth muscle cells.
   d. sphinctor muscles.

   Reference: p. 69

10. Persistent activation of a receptor leads to:

    a. increased sensitivity to the activating agent.

    *b. gradual loss of sensitivity to the activating agent.

    c. abrupt hypersensitivity to the activating agent.

    d. hypersensitivity to the activating agent if it is removed and reintroduced.

    Reference: p. 67

11. The term "downregulation" refers to:

    *a. a decrease in the number of available receptor sites

    b. an increase in the number of receptor cells.

    c. persistant receptor antagonism.

    d. a change in the response of the receptor cell itself to the activator.

    Reference: p. 68

12. Which statement best describes the action of drugs that affect central neuronal function?

    a. The drugs are singular and predictable in action.

    *b. Many drugs affect both central and peripheral nervous systems.

    c. The drugs affect a person's somatic system, but behavior patterns are not affected significantly.

    d. Most drugs elicit either hyperactive behavior or cause sedation.

    Reference: p. 68

13. The functions of alertness, arousal and consciousness is mediated by the:

    a. Limbic system

    *b. Reticular activating system

    c. Basal ganglia

    d. Thalamus

    Reference: p. 69

14. Antipsychotics or other drugs that are used to treat emotional disorders, exert a significant part of their action on the:

    *a. Limbic system

    b. Reticular activating system

    c. Basal ganglia

    d. Thalamus

    Reference: p. 69

15. Conditions such as Parkinson's Disease or Huntington's Chorea affect motor functions such as muscle tone and patterns of movement. Therefore you know that the system that is affected is the:

    a. Limbic system

    b. Reticular activation system

    *c. Basal ganglia

    d. Thalamus

    Reference: p. 68

16. Antiemetics have their action in the:

    a. Cerebrum

    *b. Medulla

    c. Cerebellum

    d. Thalamus

    Reference: p. 68

17. Water and electrolyte balance is regulated through the:

    a. thalamus

    *b. hypothalamus

    c. basal ganglia

    d. limbic system

    Reference: p. 68

18. Hormones stored in the pituitary gland are released by factors from the:

    a. thalamus

    *b. hypothalamus

    c. basal ganglia

    d. limbic system

    Reference: p. 68

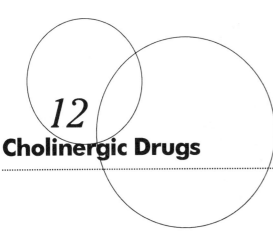

12
Cholinergic Drugs

1. Cholinergic, or cholinomimetic, drugs produce the same physiologic affect as:

   a. norepinephrine

   *b. acetylcholine

   c. choline

   d. histamine

   Reference: p. 70

2. The action of "irreversible" cholinesterase inhibitors is reversed only by:

   a. destruction of the cholinesterase enzyme, thus freeing any bound enzymes.

   b. destruction of the bond between the cholinesterase enzyme and the enzyme with which it is bound.

   *c. synthesis of new enzyme material that is unbound with cholinesterase enzyme.

   d. reduction of the activity of the cholinesterase enzyme.

   Reference: p. 70

3. Acetylcholine given as a drug has little clinical usefulness because:

   *a. it is rapidly hydrolyzed and has a short, non specific duration of action.

   b. it is slowly hydrolyzed but action is non specific.

   c. it is rapidly hydrolyzed and has limited effects upon the CNS.

   d. it is slowly hydrolyzed and has long-term action upon the CNS.

   Reference: p. 70

4. Which statement best describes the action of Miochol?

   a. The pupil is dilated, and the eye is adjusted for near vision.

   b. The pupil is dilated and the eye is adjusted for far vision.

   *c. The pupil is constricted and the eye is adjusted for near vision.

   d. The pupil is constricted and the eye is adjusted for far vision.

   Reference: p. 70

5. The action of the cholinomimetic drugs that relieve the symptoms of glaucoma is:

   a. relaxation of the ciliary muscle.

   b. dilation of the pupil.

   *c. contraction of the ciliary muscle.

   d. paralysis of the ciliary muscle.

   Reference: p. 70

6. Some cholinergic drugs are useful for treating nonobstructive urinary retention. One of these drugs is:

   a. Miostat

   b. Pilocarpine

   * c. Urecholine

   d. Habitrol

   Reference: p. 71

7. The presence of some disease states are contraindications for the use of the cholinergic, bethanechol (Urecholine). These include:

   a. Urinary retention.

   *b. Asthma.

   c. Hypertension.

   d. Tachycardia.

   Reference: p. 71

8. In event of a hypersensitive reaction or cholinergic crisis, a drug that should be available at all times as an antidote is:

   a. Quinidine.

   b. Procainamide.

   *c. Atropine Sulfate.

   d. Lidocaine.

   Reference: p. 72

9. Nursing actions that are appropriate after administration of bethanechol (Urecholine) include:

a. Frequent blood pressure checks.

b. Close monitoring of CBC and HB.

c. Frequent assessment for hepatic symptoms.

*d. Assessment for pulmonary edema.

Reference: p. 72

10. When giving carbachol (Isopto Carbachol), it is important to monitor the patient for:

a. redness, irritation of the sclerae.

b. urticaria or erythema.

*c. extreme salivation.

d. constipation.

Reference: p.72

11. The effects of cholinergic drugs on the eye include:

a. mitosis

*b. miosis

c. cycloplegia

d. mydriasis

Reference: p. 73

12. Pilocarpine has been ordered for your patient for treatment of his glaucoma. You take his history, keeping in mind that some health problems indicate caution in giving this drug. These problems include:

*a. Heart block

b. Hypertension

c. Ileus

d. Arteriosclerosis

Reference: p. 73

13. The chief therapeutic action of pilocarpine upon the eye causes:

a. relaxation of the ciliary muscle

*b. contraction of the ciliary muscle

c. dilation of the pupil

d. paralysis of the ciliary muscle

Reference: p. 73

14. The cholinesterase inhibitory effects of neostigmine causes:

*a. prolongation of the action of acetylcholine

b. blockage of the action of acetylcholine

c. increase in the uptake of acetylcholine

d. depression of production of acetylcholine

Reference: p. 74

15. A cholenergic drug that has proven to be useful in the treatment of myasthenia gravis is:

a. demecarium (Humorsol).

b. physostigmine (Eserine Sulfate).

*c. neostigmine (Prostigmin)

d. echothiophate iodide (Phospholine Iodide)

Reference: p. 75

16. Cholinergics are effective in the treatment of myasthenia gravis because they prolong the effects of:

a. norepinephrine.

b. serotonin.

c. histamine.

*d. acetylcholine.

Reference: p. 76

17. Symptoms of cholinergic overdosage include:

a. tachycardia, hypertension.

*b. excessive salivation, muscle weakness.

c. lethargy, coma.

d. nystagmus, urinary retention.

Reference: p. 76

18. In teaching your patient about nicotine gum, you would tell him/her all of the following except:

a. "The dose of nicotine is progressively lower with the use of the three-stage patches."

b. "It is common to develop a sore throat with the use of the gum."

c. "As your use of nicotine decreases, dosage requirements of other drugs that you take may change."

*d. "Insulin dosage may need to be increased as nicotine levels decrease in the body."

Reference: p. 74

19. Adverse effects of cholinergics upon the GI system include:

a. Ileus and distention

*b. Anorexia and diarrhea

c. Constipation and fecal impaction

d. Diverticulosis and fever

Reference: p. 76

20. A cholinergic drug that has proven useful in the treatment of the mild dementia of early Alzheimer's Disease is:

*a. Tacrine

b. Amantadine

c. Aldomet

d. Haldol

Reference: p. 82

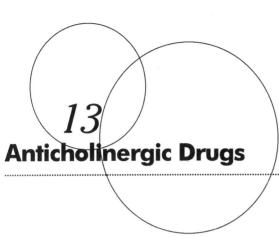

13
Anticholinergic Drugs

1. The following statement best describes the general action of anticholinergic drugs:

   a. Anticholinergic drugs combine with acetylcholine, producing a non-reactive substance.

   *b. Anticholinergic drugs block the action of acetylcholine at the cholinergic receptor site.

   c. Anticholinergic drugs depress the synthesis of acetylcholine at the preganglionic synapse.

   d. Anticholinergic drugs suppress the uptake of acetylcholine at preganglionic synapses.

   Reference: p. 85

2. The anticholinergic drugs are divided into three groups because of their specific actions upon these three areas:

   a. Cholinergic, adrenergic, and noradrenergic endings.

   b. Presynaptic, synaptic, and postsynaptic nerve endings.

   *c. Muscarinic, nicotinic, and N II receptor sites.

   d. MAO, COMT, and ACT in prejunctional nerve endings.

   Reference: p. 85

3. A major problem with the use of the anticholinergic, naturally occuring, belladona alkaloids is:

   a. The drugs have a very narrow range of action at the receptor sites.

   b. The toxicity of the drugs make therapeutic dosages difficult to achieve.

   c. The drugs must be given parenterally as they are not readily absorbed po.

   *d. A wide range of side effects occur when the drugs are used therapeutically.

   Reference: p. 85

4. What statement best describes the action of antispasmodic tertiary amines?

   a. Their central effects are minimal.

   *b. They directly act upon GI smooth muscle.

   c. They decrease the flow of gastric acid.

   d. They are effective cholinergic blockers.

Reference: p. 85

5. Emma Brown is going on a boat trip and wishes to use a scopolamine patch to avoid seasickness. Which health problem would lead you to advise her against this?

   *a. Narrow angle glaucoma

   b. Urinary frequency and urgency

   c. Persistent heart block

   d. Frequent diarrhea

   Reference: p. 90

6. Although Mrs. Brown should not wear the scopolamine patch, Mr. Smith is able to do so. You advise him concerning the possibility of adverse reactions to this drug. Side effects of scopolamine include all except:

   a. blurred vision

   b. tachycardia

   c. insommnia

   *d. diarrhea

   Reference: p. 90

7. Mr. Smith is also taking an over-the-counter antihistamine. The effect of this medication on scopolamine may be to:

   a. Increase its therapeutic effects.

   *b. Increase its side effects.

   c. Interfere with the therapeutic effects of the drug.

   d. It will have no effect on the drug.

   Reference: p. 91

8. You will need to educate Mr. Smith on the use of the scopolamine patch. As it is an anti-cholinergic, your teaching will include all except:

   a. He is to avoid the use of other over the counter preparations.

   b. He should be careful when engaging in physical activity, because antimuscarinic agents can impair coordination.

c. He may experience dry mouth and constipation.

*d. He may be bothered by excessive salivation and diarrhea.

Reference: p. 92

9. Anticholinergic drugs compete with acetylcholine at muscarinic sites in the autonomic nervous system. Systems affected include all except:

a. the eye.

b. the respiratory system

c. the urinary tract

*d. the musculo-skeletal system

Reference: pgs. 85–86

10. The effects of anticholinergics upon the eye includes:

a. meiosis

b. mitosis

*c. cycloplegia

d. tearing

Reference: p. 86

11. The effects of anticholinergics upon the respiratory system include:

a. bronchoconstriction

*b. bronchodilation

c. increased secretion

d. tachypnea

Reference: p. 86

12. The effects of anticholinergics upon the G. I. system include:

a. hypermotility

b. hyperacidity

c. diarrhea

*d. constipation

Reference: p. 86

13. Scopolamine is used preoperatively to:

a. increase the sedative properties of the other medications given preoperatively

b. facilitate anesthesia, thereby requiring lower doses of anesthetics.

*c. dry the respiratory secretions caused by anesthesia during surgery.

d. decrease the length of time of the action of anesthetics, therefore facilitating postanesthetic recovery time.

Reference: p. 86

14. Ganglionic blocking agents are often used to produce hypotension in certain circumstances, such as during surgery. Because of the resulting parasympathetic blockade, a problem that you need to assess for in these postoperative patients is:

*a. ileus and urinary retention.

b. diaphoresis and rebound hypertension.

c. bronchoconstriction and increased secretion.

d. increased G.I. motility and diarrhea.

Reference: p. 93

15. Your patient is taking Inversine after treatment with other antihypertensive drugs have failed. It is important that you teach her:

a. to take the medication after meals if dysphagia occurs.

*b. to avoid standing up suddenly.

c. to decrease her salt intake.

d. that bulk laxatives are useful for the treatment of drug induced constipation.

Reference: p. 92

16. Trimethaphan (Arfonad) is used in the treatment of:

a. chronic hypertension.

b. Addison's disease.

c. hepatitis

*d. hypertensive emergencies.

Reference: p. 94

17. Contraindications to the use of trimethaphan (Arfonad) include:

*a. anemia.

b. glaucoma.

c. myasthenia gravis.

d. porphyruria.

Reference: p. 94

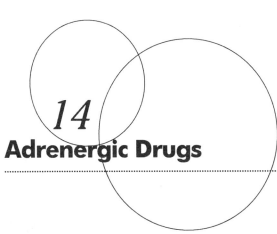

14
Adrenergic Drugs

1. Adrenergic drugs produce physiologic responses that mimic those of the:

   a. central nervous system.

   *b. sympathetic nervous system.

   c. parasympathetic nervous system.

   d. somatic nervous system.

   Reference: p. 96

2. The three naturally occurring principal adrenergic drugs include all except:

   *a. hyoscyamine sulfate

   b. epinephrine.

   c. norepinephrine.

   d. dopamine.

   Reference: p. 96

4. The hormone secreted in times of stress is:

   a. dopamine.

   b. tyramine.

   *c. epinephrine.

   d. norepinephrine.

   Reference: p. 96

4. The three major endogenous catecholamines that serve as neurotransmitters and modulators of the sympathetic nervous system include:

   a. tyramine, monamine, and serotonin.

   *b. epinephrine, norepinephrine, and dopamine.

   c. propantheline, trimethapan, and pancuronium.

   d. neostigmine, physostigmine, and pralidoxime.

   Reference: p. 96

5. The therapeutic indications for the use of catecholamines are based upon three actions of these substances. These actions are:

   *a. cardiac stimulation, bronchodilation, and vasoconstriction.

   b. cardiac depression, bronchodilation, and vasoconstriction.

   c. cardiac stimulation, bronchoconstriction and vasoconstriction.

   d. cardiac stimulation, bronchodilation and vasodilation.

   Reference: p. 97

6. Epinephrine is useful because of its activation of alpha and beta-adrenergic receptor sites. Activation of these sites causes:

   *a. peripheral vasoconstriction.

   b. decrease in heart rate.

   c. decrease in blood glucose.

   d. CNS stimulation.

   Reference: p. 97

7. An important use of epinephrine is:

   a. in the second stage of labor to enhance progress.

   *b. to restore cardiac action in the case of arrest.

   c. to lower blood pressure in hypertensive crisis.

   d. to speed recovery from anesthesia.

   Reference: p. 97

8. Epinephrine is contraindicated in:

   a. hypotensive states.

   b. allergic and anaphylactic states.

   *c. severe hypertensive crisis.

   d. nasal congestion.

   Reference: p. 97

9. An important consideration for the diabetic patient who is taking Epifrin or Eppy/N for glaucoma is that:

   a. insulin or oral hypoglycemic requirements may be decreased.

   b. epinephrine may cause vascular complications of diabetes because of vasoconstriction.

   c. the cardiac effects of epinephrine are intensified by poorly controlled hyperglycemia.

*d. epinephrine may induce hyperglycemia, increasing insulin or oral hypoglycemic requirements.
Reference: pgs. 97—98

10. The use of levarterenol (Levophed) is contraindicated in the presence of:
    a. Tachycardia.
    b. Hypotension
    *c. Hypovolemic shock.
    d. Hypoclycemia.
    Reference: p. 100

11. The most important nursing intervention during the administration of levarterenol (Levophed) is to:
    a. keep the patient warm.
    b. give with normal saline.
    *c. monitor vital signs q 2-5 minutes.
    d. administer with oxytocics.
    Reference: p. 100

12. An important drug to have available to treat possible bradycardia during administration of levarterenol (Levophed) is:
    a. propranolol.
    *b. atropine.
    c. prostigmine.
    d. adrenalin.
    Reference: p. 101

13. Renal perfusion needs to be assessed frequently during administration of levarterenol (Levophed). This is best accomplished by:
    a. serum creatinine studies on a daily basis.
    *b. urinary output recording on an hourly basis.
    c. daily weights.
    d. careful assessment for edema on each shift.
    Reference: p. 101

14. The use of dopamine (Intropin) is contraindicated in:
    *a. ventricular arrhythmias.
    b. poor renal function.
    c. bradycardia.
    d. heart block.
    Reference: p. 101

15. Decreased vasopressor effects may be seen if dopamine (Intropin) is given with:
    a. triclyclic antidepressants.
    b. MAO inhibitors.
    c. antihistamine.

*d. pheothiazine derivatives.
Reference: p. 102

16. The drug that is commonly used for Adams-Stokes syndrome and AV block is
    a. Adrenalin.
    b. Propranolol
    *c. Isuprel.
    d. Levophed.
    Reference: p. 102

17. Dobutamine (Dobutrex) is most commonly used for
    *a. short-term treatment of acute heart failure.
    b. arrhythmias associated with tachycardia.
    c. treatment of coronary artery disease.
    d. long-term treatment of hypertension.
    Reference: p. 104

18. Interaction of dobutamine (Dobutrex) with MAO inhibitors, tricyclic antidepressants and other sympathomimetics causes:
    a. cardiac dysrhythmias.
    *b. hypertension.
    c. bradycardia.
    d. hypotension.
    Reference: p. 105

19. The primary action of sympathomimetic vasopressor amines (Wyamine, Aramine, Vasoxyl) is:
    a. enhancement of cardiac contractility.
    b. overall peripheral vasodilation.
    c. skeletal muscle relaxation.
    *d. systemic vasoconstriction.
    Reference: p. 105

20. Sympathomimetic vasopressor amines are useful for the treatment of:
    a. long term treatment of congestive heart failure.
    b. short term treatment of heart block.
    *c. hypotension secondary to spinal anesthesia.
    d. hypertension due to renal failure.
    Reference: p. 105

21. Some people develop tolerance to mephentermine (Wyamine). In order to detect this effect the correct nursing action would be to:
    a. give increasingly large doses to adjust for the tolerance.
    b. give more frequent doses to maintain blood levels of the drug.

*c. evaluate your patient's response to repeated injections.

d. change the route of administration to enhance absorption.

Reference: p. 106

22. Before giving mephentermine (Wyamine), what steps should be taken for safe administration?

a. Correction of hyperthyroidism.

*b. Correction of hypovolemia.

c. Regulation of any cardiac dysrhythmias.

d. Correction of any electrolyte imbalances.

Reference: p. 106

23. The "rebound effect" from prolonged use of adrenergic decongestant nasal sprays such as Neosynephrine nasal spray often leads to:

a. mucosal irritation.

b. prolonged mucosal dryness.

*c. chronic "runny nose."

d. cardiac response.

Reference: p. 108

24. Dipivefrin (or Propine) is a soluble prodrug of epinephrine. Therefore you know that all statements are true except:

a. Dipivefrin is converted to epinephrine instillation into the eye.

*b. The action of dipivefrin causes fewer side effects than epinephrine.

c. Dipivefrin causes miosis and cycloplegia.

d. Narrow angle glaucoma is a contraindication to the use of dipivefrin.

Reference: p. 110

25. Sympathomimetic agents such as ephedrine are used as bronchodilators. In addition to this response, other effects of this drug include:

*a. contraction of the urinary spincter.

b. urinary muscle contraction.

c. relaxation of the urinary spinctors.

d. meiosis.

Reference: p. 112

26. A contraindication to the use of ephedrine is:

a. the presence of COPD.

*b. severe CAD.

c. a history of depression.

d. the presence of thyroid disease.

Reference: p. 112

27. Your patient has been taking ephedrine for a number of months for the treatment of his narcolepsy. He tells you that he is not experiencing as much relief as he did when he first began taking the drug. Your advice to him is to:

a. consult with his health care provider in order to have his dosage increased.

b. check the expiration date of his medication-the "shelf life" is very short.

c. change the route of administration to enhance the absorption of the drug.

*d. institue a drug-free interval after consultation with his health care provider.

Reference: p. 114

28. The chief advantage in the use of Bronkephrine, a beta 2 activator, is:

a. there are fewer urinary tract effects.

b. ototoxic effects are decreased.

*c. cardiac response is minimal.

d. pressor effects are not as pronounced.

Reference: p. 114

29. A major problem with the use of isoxsuprine (Vasodilan) and other sympathomimetic beta 2 agonists is that:

a. constriction of vascular capillary beds pulls circulation away from the periphery.

b. peripheral vasoconstriction decreases blood supply to vital organs.

c. rebound hypertension is a problem after prolonged therapy.

*d. peripheral vasodilation shunts blood supply away from vital organs.

Reference: p. 116

30. An important nursing intervention for a patient taking Vasodilan is:

a. repeated checks of capillary refill.

b. frequent checks for a positive Homan's sign.

*c. orthostatic blood pressure checks.

d. baseline audiometry to detect ototoxicity.

Reference: p. 116

31. Yutopar (Ritodrine) is primarily used for:

a. hypertensive crisis.

b. bronchial asthma.

*c. preterm labor.

d. eclampsia.

Reference: p. 117

32. A major problem found with the use of phenyl-
    propanolamine as an anoretic is that:

    a. it may cause a too-rapid weight loss.

    b. it can cause a hypotensive effect.

    c. it has a high potential for abuse.

    *d. it can cause tachycardia.

    Reference: p. 118

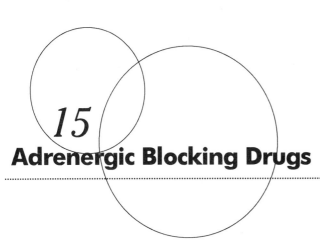

15
Adrenergic Blocking Drugs

1. The action of adrenergic blocking agents is to:
   a. mimic the effects of acetylcholine.
   b. block the action of acetylcholine
   c. mimic the stimulation of sympathetic neurons.
   *d. antagonize the actions of sympathetic neuro-transmitters.
   Reference: p. 119

2. Nonselective alpha blockers act primarily upon:
   a. skeletal striated muscle.
   b. exocrine glandular tissue.
   *c. vascular smooth muscle.
   d. nonvascular smooth muscle.
   Reference: p. 119

3. The action of alpha adrenergic blocking agents may result in:
   *a. tachycardia and hypotension.
   b. bronchospasm and tachycardia.
   c. urinary retention and hypertension.
   d. hallucinations and seizures.
   Reference: p. 119

4. The alpha adrenergic blocking agent, phenoxyben-zamine (Dibenzyline) is useful in treating:
   a. certain types of heart block.
   b. bronchoconstriction in COPD.
   *c. symptoms of pheochromocytoma.
   d. manifestations of renal insufficiency.
   Reference: p. 119

5. Phenoxybenzamine (Dibenzyline) 10mg bid po has been ordered for your patient. Your teaching includes the statement:
   a. "Your blood pressure may go up while you are taking this medication."
   *b. "Take this medication with food to minimize side effects."
   c. "You may have some respiratory symptoms when you first take this, but they will go away."

   d. "Do not take this medication with diary products."
   Reference: p. 119

6. Your patient's IV Levophed has infiltrated. Your action is to:
   a. elevate the affected arm.
   b. apply warm compresses to the affected area and inject the area with saline.
   c. apply cool compresses to the affected area and inject with dobutamine.
   *d. apply warm compresses to the affected area and inject with regitine.
   Reference: p. 120

7. Which condition would be a contraindication for the use of Regitine?
   a. Pheochromocytoma.
   b. Coronary Artery Disease.
   *c. Myocardial Infarction.
   d. Addison's Disease.
   Reference: p. 121

8. The effects of phentolamine (Regitine) persist for how long after IV injection?
   *a. 15 minutes.
   b. 30 minutes.
   c. one hour.
   d. four hours.
   Reference: p. 121

9. A valuable use of beta-adrenergic receptor blockers is to:
   a. increase the heart rate in the presence of 2nd and 3rd degree heart block.
   b. reduce the incidence of bronchospasm in ARDS.
   c. increase the peripheral blood flow in Reynauld's Disease.
   *d. slow cardiac rate and decrease contractility in tachyarrhythmias.
   Reference: p. 122

10. The action of the beta blockers in the eye results in:

    a. mitosis

    b. increased production of aqueous humor.

    c. hyperemia.

    *d. reduced production of aqueous humor.

    Reference: p. 123

11. Before starting your patient on the beta-blocking agent that was ordered for him, it is important that you these perimeters:

    *a. The presence of edema and body weight.

    b. Periodontal examination.

    c. Reflexes and muscle strength.

    d. Opthalmic examination.

    Reference: p. 124

12. Your patient has just been diagnosed with glaucoma and the physician has ordered timolol (Timoptic) opthalmic drops. As you do your assessments before initiating this therapy, what in his history would alert you to question the order?

    a. Seizures.

    b. Alcoholism.

    *c. Bronchial asthma.

    d. Pheochromocytoma.

    Reference: p. 126

13. Your patient is being treated for angina with propranolol (Inderol) 40mg qid po. It is important to instruct your patient:

    a. "Take this medication on an empty stomach as food interferes with its absorption."

    b. "You may become very sleepy while you are taking this medication; do not drive."

    c. "If you experience any disturbances in hearing, let your doctor know right away."

    *d. "Do not stop taking this medication abruptly, the dosage must be decreased gradually if it is discontinued."

    Reference: p. 126

14. Mr. Brown has been admitted to your unit with atrial flutter and esmolol (Brevibloc) IV has been ordered. Shortly after you start his infusion, you note that his heart rate has dropped to 42 bpm. What medication do you want to have on hand as you notify his physician of this development?

    a. Lopressor.

    b. Dilantin.

    *c. Atropine.

    d. Lidocaine.

16
Antihistamine and Antiserotonin agents

1. Antihistamines are best known for their H_1 receptor antagonistic effects. In contrast, the H_2 blockers primarily affect the:

   a. columnar cells of the respiratory system, causing bronchoconstriction.

   b. smooth muscle structures of the vascular system, causing vasoconstriction.

   c. cardiac muscle cells, causing increased contractility.

   *d. gastric parietal cells, causing reduced HCL secretion.

   Reference: p. 128

2. H_1 antagonists are most effective in the treatment of:

   *a. urticaria.

   b. contact dermatitis.

   c. bronchial asthma.

   d. anaphylactic reactions.

   Reference: p. 129

3. Bruce Evans, a 72 year old man, has developed allergy problems that cause intense pruritis. He is given trimeprazine (Temaril) for the relief of his symptoms. Because of his age, as you take his history you need to be particularly alert to health problems common to older people that are contraindications for the use of histamine blockers. These problems include:

   a. a history of pheochromocytoma.

   b. gall bladder disease and diabetes.

   c. vascular problems or cardiac arrhythmias.

   *d. glaucoma or bladder obstruction.

   Reference: p. 132

4. Before he begins to take his antihistamine, your instructions to Mr. Evans include the statement:

   *a. "Do not use over the counter medications while taking this antihistamine."

   b. "Take your antihistamine between meals if GI irritation occurs."

   c. "This medication can be taken safely for long periods of time."

   d. "This particular antihistamine has few side effects."

   Reference: p. 133

5. Extrapyramidial symptoms (Parkinsonian reactions, sedation) are significant adverse reactions to watch for when giving:

   a. diphenhydramine(Benadryl)

   *b. trimeprazine (Temaril)

   c. astemizole (Hismanil)

   d. terfenadine (Seldane)

   Reference: p. 132

6. Anticholinergic effects of phenothiazines such as Temaril are intensified by:

   *a. MAO inhibitors, tricyclic antidepressants, thiazide diuretics.

   b. antiarrhythmics, antihypertensives, aminoglycosides.

   c. alkylating agents, barbiturates, beta-blockers.

   d. cardiac glycosides, corticosteriods, narcotics.

   Reference: p. 133

7. Important assessments for the nurse to perform before giving the first dose of a phenothiazine-type antihistamine are:

   a. skin turgor, cardiac rhythm and rate.

   b. muscle spasticity, coordination.

   *c. reflexes, orthostatic blood pressure.

   d. hearing difficulties, fluid status.

   Reference: p. 133

8. Your patient, Mr. Smith is being treated for his gastric ulcer with cimetidine (Tagamet). You tell him that the most important action of H2 antagonists is to:

   a. decrease gastric motility.

   *b. inhibit gastric acid secretion.

34

c. increase the absorbant action of the gastric mucosa.

d. enhance the action of calcium channel blockers.

Reference: p. 137

9. A common use of Benadryl is:

a. Treatment of seasonal allergic rhinitis.

b. Ongoing treatment of vertigo.

c. Intitial treatment of pruritus.

*d. Adjunctive therapy of anaphylactic reactions.

Reference: p. 131

10. Cimetidine(Tagamet) interacts with:

a. Aminoglycosides.

b. Sulfonamides.

*c. Beta blockers.

d. Anticoagulants.

Reference: p. 138

11. Ergotamine is useful for vascular and migrane headaches because of its action of:

*a. vasoconstriction.

b. vasodilation.

c. muscle relaxation.

d. oxytocic effects.

Reference: p. 139

12. Meclizine is used in the treatment of:

*a. Motion sickness.

b. Insomnia.

c. Allergic disorders.

d. Parkinsonism.

Reference: p. 131

13. The antihistamine commonly used for preoperative and obstetrical sedation is:

a. Terfenadine (Seldane).

b. Pyrilamine (Dormarex).

*c. Promethazine (Phenergan).

d. Triprolidine (Actidil).

Reference: p. 131

14. Important symptoms of an adverse reaction to ergotamine are:

a. cardiac arrhythemias.

b. nausea and vomiting.

c. petechiae and easy bruising.

*d. tingling in the extremities.

Reference: p. 140

15. A drug used for prophylaxis of migrane attacks is:

a. Dihydroergotamine (D.H.E. 45).

*b. Methysergide (Sansert).

c. Rantidine (Zantac).

d. Ergotamine (Ergostat).

Reference: p. 140

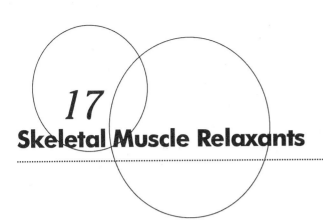

17
Skeletal Muscle Relaxants

1. The immediate muscle flaccidity caused by nondepolarizing muscle relaxants make these drugs useful for:

   a. treatment for muscle spasticity.

   b. minimizing the effects of myasthenia gravis.

   c. treatment of skeletal muscle injury.

   *d. muscle paralysis during general anesthesia.

   Reference: p. 143

2. Your patient, James Brown is on a ventilator after a head injury. Doxacurium (Numorax) has been ordered to facilitate the mechanical ventilation needed. As the margin of safety for this medication is narrow, you want on hand as an antidote:

   a. Timolol

   b. Esmolol

   *c. Levarterenol

   d. Ritodrine

   Reference: p. 145

3. Your patient, Mr. Brown is on a *depolarizing* blocker, succinylcholine. The medication that is *contraindicated for overdosage is:*

   a. vasopressors (levarterenol)

   *b. cholinesterase inhibitors (edrophonium)

   c. beta-blockers (timolol)

   d. corticosteroids (depo-medrol)

   Reference: p. 144

4. You review Mr. Brown's history before starting doxacurium. You note that he has had extensive lab work. Findings that would contraindicate the use of nondepolarizing blockers include:

   a. anemia

   b. high creatinine levels

   *c. electrolyte imbalance

   d. high BUN

   Reference: p. 144

5. Your important baseline physical assessment parameters that are necessary to detect possible future adverse reactions to doxacurium are:

   a. pupillary reactions

   b. audiometry

   *c. liver palpation

   d. palpation of the kidneys

   Reference: p. 144

6. Nursing actions that are important for the patient who is being given doxacurium include all except:

   *a. assessment of the patient's intake and output on an hourly basis.

   b. monitoring for wheezing, urticaria, bronchospasm.

   c. turning frequently to prevent skin breakdown.

   d. frequent vital signs to detect parasympathomimetic stimulation.

   Reference: p. 144

7. Which of the skeletal muscle relaxants is also used for the treatment of malignant hyperthermia?

   a. Succinylcholine (Anectine)

   b. Baclofen (Lioresal)

   c. Pancuronium Reference: avulon)

   *d. Dantrolene (Dantrium)

   Reference: p. 150

8. Direct acting skeletal muscle relaxants work differently from centrally acting muscle relaxants by:

   a. acting on spinal cord motor reflex pathways.

   b. its action on smooth muscles.

   *c. directly affecting skeletal muscles.

   d. direct action on the Cerebellum.

   Reference: p. 150

9. Your education for your patient who is taking dantrolene (Dantrium) includes this statement:

   a. "You may be bothered with constipation while you are taking this medication."

b. "Be careful about taking antibiotics because certain antibiotics block the metabolism of skeletal muscle relaxants."

c. "Skeletal muscle relaxants may cause hypotension-be careful about standing up suddenly."

*d. "You may have urinary problems while taking this type of medication."

Reference: p. 151

10. You tell your patient who is taking dantrolene (Dantrium) to be sure to inform his doctor if all of the following occur except:

a. yellowing of the eyes.

b. skin rash

*c. blurred vision

d. easy bruising

Reference: p. 150

11. As you read the history and physical in the chart, what fact alerts you that your patient is a poor candidate for Dantrium therapy?

a. The presence of muscle spasticity following a CVA.

b. A history of renal disease.

c. Prior history of cardiac failure.

*d. He is 55 years old.

Reference: p. 150

12. Dantrolene (Dantrium) interacts with:

*a. Estrogens.

b. Antiacids.

c. Aminoglycosides

d. Sulfonamides.

Reference: p. 150

13. The best skeletal muscle relaxant for your patient with a strained tendon is:

a. peripherally acting muscle relaxants.

b. antidepolarizing blockers.

c. depolarizing blockers.

*d. centrally acting muscle relaxants.

Reference: p. 150

14. A significant problem with the centrally acting skeletal muscle relaxants used for muscle injuries is:

a. hepatic damage.

b. extrapyramidial reactions.

*c. sedative effects.

d. hypotensive effects.

Reference: p. 151

15. Cyclobenzaprine (Flexeril) interacts with:

a. Anticoagulants.

*b. MAO inhibitors.

c. Anticonvulsants.

d. Cardiac glycosides.

Reference: p. 152

16. Important lab studies for your patient while taking Metaxalone (Skelaxin) include:

a. Renal function tests.

b. CBC and differentials.

c. Thyroid function tests.

*d. Liver function studies.

Reference: p. 152

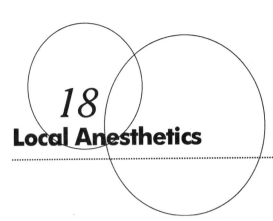

18
Local Anesthetics

1. The effects of local anesthetics are produced by:
   a. inhibition at the synapse.
   *b. blockage of nerve transmission.
   c. increased nerve depolarization.
   d. paralysis of nerve roots.
   Reference: p. 156

2. A local anesthetic combined in rectal ointments that is slowly absorbed from mucous membranes and is used to control rectal pain is:
   a. benoxinate and sodium fluorescein.
   b. bupivacaine.
   c. etidocaine.
   *d. benzocaine.
   Reference: p. 157

3. A patient admitted to an outpatient gastrointestinal laboratory a gastroscopy is given dyclonine, a local surface anesthetic. The patient may be safely discharged when she/he:
   a. begins to cough productively.
   b. is able to verbalize personal needs.
   c. complains of a "sore throat"
   *d. has a gag reflex and can swallow.
   Reference: p. 157

4. An expected reaction to the epinephrine added to a local anesthetic to decrease systemic absorption is:
   a. sleepiness and lethargy.
   *b. slight elevation in blood pressure.
   c. a decrease in respirations.
   d. a decrease in blood pressure.
   Reference: p. 159

5. Mary Merkit is scheduled to receive the epidural anesthetic tetracaine Reference: ontocaine) during labor. All of the following are correct in regard to this drug *except*:
   a. it should not be used if there is fetal bradycardia.
   b. hypotension is a contraindication to its use.
   *c. its effects are short acting, lasting 60 minutes.
   d. it is contraindicated if placenta previa exists.
   Reference: pgs. 158—159

6. Nursing assessment of the patient following spinal anesthesia should include close monitoring for:
   a. difficulty in speaking.
   *b. low blood pressure.
   c. skin color changes.
   d. elevated temperature.
   Reference: p. 159

7. Lidocaine hydrochloride (Xylocaine) with epinephrine is to be used as local anesthetic for a patient who is having surgery for the removal of an ingrown toenail. Because of a possible drug-drug interaction resulting in severe hypertension, its use would be contraindicated if the individual is taking:
   a. cholinergics.
   *b. MAO inhibitors.
   c. narcotic agonists.
   d. oral hypoglycemics.
   Reference: p. 160

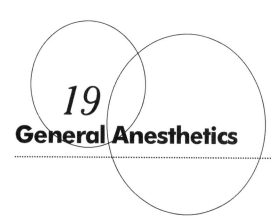

19
General Anesthetics

1. The nurse is preparing to administer atropine sulfate, an anticholinergic agent, to Janice Vorhees who is scheduled for a radical neck dissection. The correct explanation given by the nurse as to the drugs effects is:

   a. "It will help control your postoperative pain."

   b. "You will feel less anxious and much calmer."

   *c. "It will reduce salivary and mucous secretions."

   d. "You will forget events occurring prior to surgery."

   Reference: p. 162

2. Succinylcholine, a neuromuscular blocking agents, is frequently given in combination with an inhalation anesthetic to:

   a. decrease postoperative vomiting.

   b. prevent heart block/bradycardia.

   *c. allow a lower dose of anesthetic.

   d. decrease postoperative pain.

   Reference: p. 163

3. Following Eve Marker's surgery for cholecystectomy she is unable to void and develops urinary retention. A drug that her physician may prescribe to help restore normal bladder function is:

   a. bisacodyl.

   *b. bethanechol.

   c. prochlorperazine .

   d. diazepam.

   Reference: p. 163

4. In a preoperative assessment of a patient, the nurse discovers the person has chronic obstructive pulmonary disease, a possible contraindication to the use of:

   a. inhalation anesthetics.

   *b. volatile liquid anesthetics.

   c. intravenous anesthetics.

   d. neutroleptanalgetic agent.

   Reference: p. 164

5. Jim McDow, age 18, received a combination of nitrous oxide and isoflurane inhalation anesthesia for an appendectomy. Postoperatively, the reaction the patient is most likely to exhibit is:

   a. an increased blood pressure.

   b. moderate nausea and vomiting.

   c. an irregular heart rhythm.

   *d. impaired motor function.

   Reference: pgs. 164—166

6. Marge MacDonald is to receive nitrous oxide for a minor surgical procedure at an outpatient surgical clinic. Health teaching by the nurse should include the following explanation:

   a. "You will go to sleep quickly but wake up very slowly."

   b. "You can drive yourself home safely right after you awaken."

   *c. "You may experience vivid dreams and hallucinations."

   d. "Abdominal distention occurs from decreased bowel activity."

   Reference: p. 164

7. All of the following are typical side-effects the nurse might observe in patients who have received inhalation anesthetic therapy *except*:

   a. impaired psychomotor function.

   b. nausea and vomiting.

   c. complaints of "being cold"/shivering.

   *d. a drastic increase in temperature.

   Reference: p. 164

8. Gene Claus develops malignant hyperthermia following surgery for a right hemicolectomy. The drug the nurse would anticipate as being used to treat this condition is:

   *a. dantrolene IV.

   b. succinylcholine IV.

   c. morphine sulfate IV.

   d. thiopental IV.

   Reference: p. 164

9. Major advantages of intravenous barbiturates as compared to inhalation anesthetics include all of the following except:

a. rapid onset and speedy recovery.

*b. low incidence of laryngospasm.

c. little danger of arrhythmias.

d. greater patient acceptance.

Reference: p. 168

10. Connie Hines, 45 years old, has suffered extensive burn trauma. She is given ketamine (Ketalar) for a wound debridement procedure. The drug of choice to control the delirium and excitement the patient sometimes exhibits during the recovery phase from the anesthetic is:

a. a neuroleptanalgesic

b. a neuromuscular blocking agent

c. an short-acting analgesic

*d. a rapid-acting barbiturate

Reference: p. 171

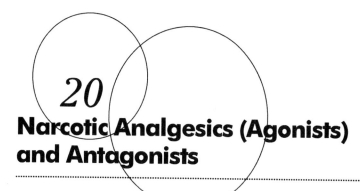

20
Narcotic Analgesics (Agonists) and Antagonists

1. Opiate analgesics are contraindicated or used cautiously in all of the following except in those patients:

    a. known to have hepatic cirrhosis.

    *b. who express a fear of drug addiction.

    c. with increased intracranial pressure.

    d. with undiagnosed acute abdominal pain

    Reference: pgs. 174—180

2. The possibility of addiction to opiate analgesics would be of greatest concern to the nurse in patients experiencing:

    a. pain occurring during terminal illness from cancer.

    b. acute post-surgical pain during hospitalization.

    *c. long-term chronic pain from a back injury.

    d. pain for 3 days after a severe physical trauma.

    Reference: p. 175

3. In preparation for the removal of a patient's perineal packing following surgery for colorectal cancer, the physician prescribes morphine sulfate 10 mg IV. Prior to administering the drug the nurse should carefully assess the patient's:

    a. bowel sounds.

    *b. respiratory rate/depth.

    c. deep tendon reflexes.

    d. temperature and pulse.

    Reference: p. 176

4. A patient who is receiving a subcutaneous injection of fentanyl for severe postoperative pain asks the nurse, "How soon can I expect to experience some relief from this injection?" The nurse would correctly respond:

    *a. "Within 20 minutes."

    b. "In 35 minutes."

    c. "In 45 minutes."

    d. "In about 55 minutes."

    Reference: p. 177

5. The management of pain associated with such conditions as burn trauma, post-surgical trauma, myocardial infarction, and fractures is best accomplished with the use of:

    a. benzodiazepines.

    b. non-steroidal antiinflammatory drugs.

    c. hypnotics.

    *d. opioid derivatives.

    Reference: p. 179

6. In addition to the use of opiates for the control of pain in clinical situations they are utilized for all of the following except:

    a. to relieve persistent nonproductive cough.

    b. to relieve dyspnea associated with pulmonary edema.

    *c. to reverse edema associated with brain trauma.

    d. improve respirations of patients on ventilators.

    Reference: p. 179

7. The physician prescribes meperidine (Demerol) 75-100 mg IM every 3—4 hours PRN for pain for the first few days following the surgical repair of a femoral fracture. The nurse should plan to administer the analgesic to the patient:

    a. every 4 hours for 24 hours.

    b. with complaints of acute pain

    c. with physical signs of pain.

    *d. prior to onset of intense pain.

    Reference: p. 180

8. In the patient who is unable to speak or who is nonalert, physical signs of pain that are likely to be exhibited include all of the following except:

    a. restlessness.

    b. grimacing.

    c. tachypnea/tachycardia.

    *d. pupillary dilation.

    Reference: p. 181

9. In the patient experiencing severe pain being treated with opiate analgesics, the primary objective of nursing care is to:

a. prevent physical dependence.

b. provide comforting measures.

c. facilitate coping behavior.

*d. prevent or alleviate the pain.

Reference: pgs. 180—181

10. Following surgery for an appendectomy, a 17 year old patient's requests for the prescribed analgesic meperidine (Demerol) 75-100 mg SC every 3-4 hours for "abdominal pain" have increased in frequency over a 5 day period. An action by the nurse should be to:

a. ask the physician to increase the prescribed dosage.

*b. evaluate the patient for possible complications.

c. explain to the patient the risk of addiction..

d. give a placebo to rule out physical dependence.

Reference: p. 181

11. Because of a possible drug-to-drug interaction leading to potentiation of toxicity, narcotic analgesics should be avoided in the patient taking:

a. aminoglycoside antibiotics.

*b. MAO inhibitors.

c. aminophylline.

d. phenytoin.

Reference: p. 181

12. A patient admitted to the emergency room for suspected narcotic overdosage is given naloxone (Narcan) 0.4 mg IV. Presuming the first dose is ineffective, the nurse should plan to administer the next dose in:

*a. 2—3 minutes.

b. 5—7 minutes.

c. 9—11 minutes.

d. 13—15 minutes.

Reference: p. 182

13. A newborn infant suffering from CNS depression secondary to opiates the mother received during labor, is given naloxone (Narcan) in the delivery room. Nurses assessing the infant after admission to the newborn nursery should be particularly alert to the possibility of:

a. urinary retention.

b. paradoxical excitement.

c. rapid respiratory rate.

*d. recurrent CNS depression.

Reference: p. 183

14. An agent that is prescribed as adjunctive therapy to maintain an opioid-free state in detoxified former addicts is:

a. pentazocine.

b. naloxone.

*c. naltrexone.

d. nalbuphine.

Reference: p. 183

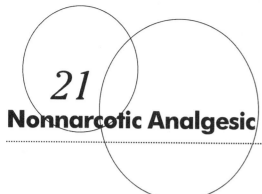

21

Nonnarcotic Analgesic and Anti-inflammatory Drugs

Kelsie Phillips, a nurse employed in an outpatient arthritis clinic is responsible for the nursing management of a variety of patients with arthritis and other rheumatoid disorders. The following are typical clinical situations she experiences.

Marita Landi is a 22 year old dancer in a Broadway musical. Following a long period of intense practice sessions she develops severe pain and inflammation in her feet/toes (metatarsophalangeal joints) and is diagnosed as having rheumatoid osteoarthritis. To control her pain and induce an antiinflammatory effect her physician prescribes high dosages of aspirin.

1. Included in the patient's teaching plan relative to taking high dosages of aspirin for rheumatoid osteoarthritis should be instructions to:

   *a. take the drug with food or after meals.

   b. stop the drug with mild gastric upset.

   c. expect weight gain from water retention.

   d. check for bloody urine at each voiding.

   Reference: p. 190

2. The nurse teaches the patient to report early signs of aspirin overdose as:

   a. epigastric distress/belching.

   b. anorexia/constipation.

   c. insomnia/anxiety.

   *d. tinnitus/hearing loss.

   Reference: p. 190

3. Because of the epigastric distress experienced with taking high dosages of aspirin, the patient asks the nurse "Why can't I just take acetaminophen (Tylenol) for my rheumatoid arthritis? An appropriate response by the nurse would be:

   *a. "It not effective in reducing joint inflammation."

   b. "It doesn't concentrate in the joints like aspirin."

   c. "It is not well absorbed by the GI tract."

   d. "In arthritic conditions it causes water retention."

   Reference: pgs. 186—189

4. The patient follows the nurse's suggestions to reduce the gastric irritation associated with taking high dosages of aspirin but continues to complain of "epigastric distress." The nurse should advise the patient to take:

   a. ancetaminophen (Tylenol).

   *b. enteric coated preparations (Ecotrin).

   c. effervescent preparations (Alka-Seltzer).

   d. buffered aspirin (Bufferin).

   Reference: p. 190

5. Drugs commonly used in the treatment of rheumatoid osteoarthritis include all of the following *except*:

   a. corticosteroids.

   b. NSAIDs.

   *c. uricosurics.

   d. pyrazolones.

   Reference: p. 191

6. It becomes apparent after 12 weeks of aspirin therapy that the pain the patient is experiencing from rheumatoid osteoarthritics is not well controlled and the physician prescribes gold therapy with aurothioglucose (Solganal) IM. To determine suitability for aurothioglucose therapy, the nurse should assess the patient's willingness to:

   a. take drugs 4-6 times a day.

   *b. commit to long term therapy.

   c. self-administer IM injections.

   d. have occasional blood and urine tests.

   Reference: p. 198

7. A laboratory value that would alert the nurse to a possible significant adverse reaction in a patient on gold therapy is:

   a. a creatinine level of less than 1.2 mg/dl

   *b. a white blood count of less than 4,000/mm^3

   c. a granulocyte count over 1,500/mm^3

   d. a serum protein level of 8 g/dl.

   Reference: p. 198

8. The patient's statements that indicates the nurse's health teaching relative to gold injections for treatment of osteoarthritis was successful is:

   a. "Right after my injections, I can get up and go home."

   b. "This medication could cause me to have tarry stools."

   *c. "It may take as several months for benefits to be felt."

   d. "I know I will need to drink a lot of water every day."

   Reference: p. 199

9. Following administration of the aurothioglucose (Solganal) deep into the gluteal muscle the nurse should:

   a. apply cold packs to the site for 20 minutes.

   b. tell the patient she will experience nausea.

   c. check her blood glucose level in 20 minutes.

   *d. instruct the patient to remain lying for 20 minutes.

   Reference: p. 199

10. A specific antidote to gold therapy that the nurse should expect to be available for use is:

    a. protamine sulfate.

    b. naloxone hydrochloride (Narcan).

    *c. dimercaprol (BAL).

    d. vitamin B$_{12}$.

    Reference: p. 199

11. Health teaching for patients on gold therapy should include informing them that a commonly experienced side effect is:

    a. lethargy.

    b. chest pain.

    c. anorexia.

    *d. skin rash.

    Reference: p. 198

12. The nurse should advise patients who are receiving aurothioglucose (Solganal) to avoid exposure to sunlight to reduce the risk of:

    a. first or second degree burns.

    b. uneven hyperpigmentation.

    *c. gold deposits in body tissues.

    d. a hypersensitivity reaction.

    Reference: p. 199

Mabel Lebam, a 69 year old housewife, is admitted to the clinic for complaints of hip and knee pain. Mrs. Lebam's drug history reveals that she takes an oral hypoglycemic, chlorpropamide (Diabenese), a beta-blocking agent, atenolol (Tenormin), a diuretic, hydrochlorthiazide, and an anticoagulant, warfarin (Coumadin). A diagnoses of "degenerative osteoarthritis" is made and the physician prescribes piroxicam (Feldene).

13. The nurse explains to the patient that the intended therapeutic effect of piroxicam (Feldene) that has been prescribed for their degenerative osteoarthritis is:

    a. to reverse joint deformities.

    b. to alter the course of the disease.

    *c. to improve joint function.

    d. to prevent joint ankylosis.

    Reference: p. 194

14. In the individual taking an NSAID, which of the following conditions reported in their past medical history indicates a possible contraindication to its use?

    a. diverticulosis

    b. hiatal hernia

    c. recurrent cholecystitis

    *d. a bleeding ulcer episode

    Reference: p. 197

15. In relation to an understanding of drug interactions with the piroxicam (Feldene), which of the statements by the patient indicates that health teaching has been successful?

    *a. "I'll take acetaminophen for a headache."

    b. "Aspirin will add to the effect this drug."

    c. "I'll take it one hour before meals with water."

    d. "If pain isn't controlled, I'll repeat the dose."

    Reference: p. 196

16. In the patient taking an NSAID and anticoagulant concurrently, the nurse would expect to monitor the:

    a. amylase level.

    b. platelet level.

    c. total albumin.

    *d. prothrombin time.

    Reference: p. 197

17. Changes in self-care the nurse should advise the patient taking chlorpropamide (Diabenese) concurrently with piroxicam (Feldene) to make is to:

    a. increase their dose of chlorpropamide

    b. check their urine for glucose

    *c. test blood glucose more frequently

    d. reduce caloric intake

    Reference: p. 197

18. Health teaching in relation to dietary intake in patients taking NSAIDS should include instruction to:

  a. increase fiber and grains.

 *b. decrease salty foods.

  c. decrease dairy products.

  d. increase citrus fruit.

  Reference: p. 197

Greg Morris, a 42 year old, slightly overweight businessman, is seen by a clinic physician for complaints of rapid onset of extreme tenderness and pain in his right ankle following a minor injury he sustained during a tennis game. The ankle appears dusky and swollen. A diagnosis of gouty arthritis is made.

19. As initial therapy for gouty arthritis, the physician prescribes colchicine 1 mg as an initial dose followed by 0.5 mg. The nurse would instruct the patient to continue to take this dose:

 *a. every 1—2 hours until his pain is relieved.

  b. daily as a preventive dose indefinitely.

  c. as a maintenance dose every 8 hours.

  d. every 4 hours during in the acute phase.

  Reference: p. 201

20. The nurse should instruct the patient who is taking colchicine to immediately report:

  a. tinnitus.

 *b. nausea, vomiting.

  c. joint stiffness.

  d. wakefulness.

  Reference: p. 202

21. In addition to taking the prescribed colchicine during the acute phase of his gouty arthritis, the patient should be instructed to do all of the following except:

  a. immobilize the affected joint.

  b. avoid tight laced high-top boots.

 *c. apply heat to the affected joint.

  e. begin a weight reduction program.

  Reference: p. 202

22. Health teaching for patients with gouty arthritis should include instructions to decrease their dietary intake of:

  a. milk, yogurt, cheese.

 *b. meat soups, liver, alcohol.

  c. bread, bran, beans.

  d. oranges, apples, prunes.

  Reference: p. 202

23. The nurse correctly explains to the patient that the allopurinol (Zyloprin) their physician has prescribed for gouty arthritis produces its effects by:

  a. inhibiting prostaglandin synthesis.

 *b. blocking uric acid production.

  c. preventing joint destruction.

  d. producing xanthine oxidase.

  Reference: p. 205

24. Following the acute phase of gouty arthritis, a patient's physician prescribes allopurinol (Zyloprim) 400 mg PO twice daily. Health teaching by the nurse should emphasize the importance of:

  a. keeping his ankle immobilized.

 *b. a fluid intake of 2-3 quarts per day.

  c. taking the drug an hour before meals.

  d. avoiding taking the drug at bedtime.

  Reference: p. 206

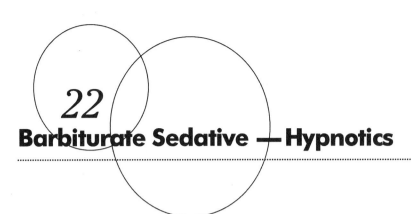

22
Barbiturate Sedative — Hypnotics

1. The most common current indication for use of barbiturates is for:

   a. hypnosis.

   b. anxiety control.

   *c. seizure control.

   d. pain control.

   Reference: p. 208

2. All of the following are associated with the long term use of barbiturates except:

   a. changes in "REM" sleep patterns.

   *b. a minimal "hangover" effect.

   c. rapid development of tolerance.

   d. convulsions with withdrawal.

   Reference: p. 208

3. The barbiturate used as adjunctive treatment for grand mal and petit mal epilepsy that produces the least amount of drowsiness is:

   a. phenobarbital.

   b. amobarbital.

   c. pentobarbital.

   *d. mephobarbital.

   Reference: p. 209

4. Sami Redd is a 70 year old female who recently lost her husband of 50 years. Because of her complaints of "wakefulness," her physician orders secobarbital sodium (Seconal) 100 mg PO at bedtime. Of the following conditions the patient reveals, the one that is a probable contraindication to the use of the drug is a history of:

   *a. liver impairment.

   b. neurosis.

   c. angina pectoris.

   d. diverticulosis.

   Reference: p. 210

5. In the patient who is taking secobarbital, a drug which is being taken concurrently that is likely to require an adjustment to increase the dosage is:

   a. a bronchodilator.

   b. an antiarrhytmic.

   *c. an anticoagulant.

   d. a vasodilator.

   Reference: p. 210

6. In relation to teaching the patient about the prescribed secobarbital, it is important to include instructions to do all of the following except:

   a. stop the usual bedtime alcholol intake.

   *b. keep the drug at the bedside.

   c. avoid taking antihistamines.

   d. change positions cautiously.

   Reference pgs. 211—212

7. A characteristic of barbiturates that accounts for the preferential use of benzodiazepines for hypnosis is:

   a. a tendency to cause hypersensitivity reactions.

   *b. a greater potential for drug dependence.

   c. a propensity for hepatotoxicity.

   d. a high incidence of delirium.

   Reference: p. 211

8. When combined with secobarbital, the drug that increases the patient's risk of injury from a fall is:

   a. amikacin.

   b. aminophylline.

   *c. furosemide.

   d. acetaminophen.

   Reference: p. 211

46

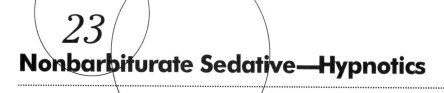

23
Nonbarbiturate Sedative—Hypnotics

1. "Anterograde amnesia," a type of short term memory loss that occurs after ingestion of a benzodiazepine drug or alcohol to induce sleep, has occurred with the use of:

   a. quazepam (Doral).

   b. estazolam Reference: roSom).

   *c. triazolam (Halcion).

   d. temazepam (Restoril).

   Reference: p. 214

2. Two days following radical mastectomy surgery, Ginny McGinnis complains of insomnia and requests a medication "to make me fall asleep." The nurse obtains an order for a benzodiazepine, flurazepam (Dalmane) 30 mg PO. A condition revealed in the patient's health history that would indicate cautious use any benzodiazepine is:

   a. epileptic seizures.

   b. peptic ulcer disease.

   *c. suicidal tendencies.

   d. diabetes mellitus.

   Reference: p. 214

3. The patient asks the nurse administering flurazepam (Dalmane) for insomnia, "How soon will the I feel the effects of the drug?" The nurse's answer is based on the knowledge that, after oral administration, sleep usually occurs:

   a. in 50-60 minutes.

   *b. in 15-45 minutes.

   c. in 5-10 minutes.

   d. immediately.

   Reference: p. 214

4. The physician orders triazolam (Halcion) for Cecil Sou, a 78 year old patient who has recently undergone a colon resection and is having difficulty fall-ing asleep. Nursing interventions should include all of the following except:

   *a. administering drug with an antacid.

   b. encouraging relaxing pre-sleep activity.

   c. limiting environmental stimuli.

   d. withholding the drug if the patient naps.

   Reference: p. 215

5. Landry Gardner, age 72, who has had a transurethral prostatectomy complains of "sleeplessness." The physician prescribes chloral hydrate PO at bedtime. The side effects is the patient is most likely to experience is:

   a. disturbed REM sleep, vivid dreams.

   *b. "hangover" effects, gastric distress.

   c. CNS depression, slowed respirations.

   d. liver and kidney impairment.

   Reference: p. 215

6. Health teaching for the patient taking chloral hydrate should include instructing the patient:

   a. to ingest the drug before a meal.

   b. to lie down immediately after taking it.

   *c. to take it with a full glass of water.

   d. to chew the capsule, swallow it with water.

   Reference: p. 216

7. In response to the patient's request for "a mild sleeping medication in the event I have trouble sleeping after I leave the hospital," the physician orders chloral hydrate. The dosage range for chloral hydrate is:

   a. 200-400 mg.

   *b. 500-1,000 mg.

   c. 1.5-2 g.

   d. 50-100 mg/kg.

   Reference: p. 215

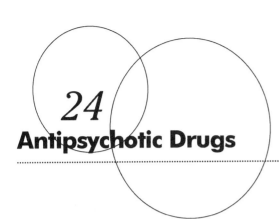

24
Antipsychotic Drugs

1. The largest and most widely used group of antipsychotic drugs are the:

   a. MAO inhibitors.

   b. benzodiazepines.

   c. tricyclic antidepressants.

   *e. phenothiazines.

   Reference: p. 221

2. A neurological syndrome associated with long term use of antipsychotic drugs characterized by involuntary abnormal muscle movements of the orofacial area (repetitive protrusion of the tongue, chewing, puffing of the cheeks, puckering of the mouth) is:

   a. Parkinsonism.

   b. akathisia.

   c. dystonia.

   *d. tardive dyskinesia.

   Reference: p. 223

3. Side effects from anticholinergic activity that are commonly experienced by the patient during the early stages of therapy with antipsychotic agents are:

   a. drowsiness, sleepiness, inattentiveness.

   b. dizziness, orthostatic hypotension.

   *c. dry mouth, blurred vision, urinary hesitancy.

   d. neck spasms, eye rolling, dysphagia.

   Reference: p. 223

4. An antipsychotic drug widely used pre- and post-operatively and for the control of nausea and vomiting is:

   *a. prochlorperazine (Compazine).

   b. chlorpromazine (Thorazine).

   c. promazine (Sparine).

   d. haloperidol (Haldol).

   Reference: p. 226

5. The nurse should help patients who are taking antipsychotic drugs understand that they must adhere to the prescribed long-term therapeutic regimen and avoid discontinuing them abruptly because:

   a. when symptoms are controlled counseling isn't needed.

   b. their addictive qualities require withdrawal sedation.

   *c. psychotic reactions might recur if they are stopped.

   d. sudden withdrawal is associated with hypertension.

   Reference: p. 228

Julianna Onrelas is a 24 year old graduate student in physics attending Pericos University. She is involved in various campus activities and has an active social life. Because she has been is unable to sit still, finds it difficult to study, and has been very argumentive and hostile towards her friends, she makes an appointment to see a psychiatrist. The psychiatrist diagnoses Julianna as being in the manic phase of a manic-depressive psychosis. The physician initially orders lithium carbonate 600 mg 3 times/day.

6. A drug taken concurrently with lithium that increases the potential for a toxic reaction to it is:

   a. an antibiotic.

   b. an H₂ receptor antagonist.

   *c. a diuretic.

   d. a multivitamin.

   Reference: p. 229

7. The nurse instructs a patient taking lithium to return to clinic for blood draws to determine serum lithium levels. Lithium toxicity is most like to occur if levels exceed:

   a. 0.5 mEq/L.

   b. 0.75 mEq/L.

   c. 1.0 mEq/L.

   *d. 1.5 mEq/L.

   Reference: p. 229

8. Health teaching for patients taking lithium should include instructions to:

a. decrease intake of salty foods.

b. increase calcium and iron intake

*c. increase daily fluid intake to 3,000 ml.

d. increase salt intake, decrease fluid intake.

Reference: p. 230

9. Health teaching for patients taking lithium should include all of the following instructions *except*:

a. record weekly weight.

*b. avoid eating aged cheeses.

c. muscle incoordination, ataxia.

d. avoid hazardous activities.

Reference: p. 230

10. During the first few weeks of lithium therapy, health teaching should include advising the patient to exercise caution in:

a. studying to excess.

*b. operating power tools.

c. playing racket ball.

d. sun bathing.

Reference: p. 230

11. After several days of lithium therapy, the patient says, "I don't know why I am taking this drug, it doesn't seem to be alleviating my symptoms!" An appropriate response by the nurse would be:

a. "You need to relax and get more rest."

b. "Make sure you stop alcohol intake."

c. "It is likely that you need a higher dose."

*d. "Effects usually occur in 1—2 weeks."

Reference: p. 230

12. A common side effect of lithium therapy that the patient may experience in the early phase of treatment is:

*a. fine hand tremors

b. slurred speech.

c. incontinence.

d. slowed heart rate.

Reference: p. 229

13. The most effective agent for controlling the severe motor and phonic tics (lack of motor coordination, vulgar language and barking sounds) in patients with Gilles de la Tourette's syndrome is:

a. droperidol (Inapsine).

*b. pimozide (Orap).

c. chlorprothixene (Taractan).

d. fluphenazine rolixin).

Reference: p. 229

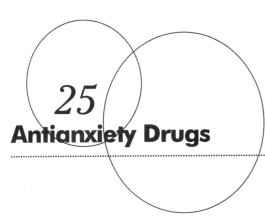

25
Antianxiety Drugs

1. Benzodiazepines are widely used as antianxiety agents because of their effectiveness and because:

    a. tolerance does not develop over time.

    b. the need for counseling is eliminated.

    *c. of the low incidence of adverse reactions.

    d. alcohol can be safely consumed with them.

    Reference: p. 233

2. A drug commonly used to control acute recurrent convulsive episodes (status epilepticus) is:

    a. midazolam (Versed) IV.

    b. chlordiazepoxide (Librium) IM.

    *c. diazepam (Valium) IV.

    d. hydroxyzine (Vistaril) IM.

    Reference: p. 235

3. Health teaching for the patient taking benzodiazepines includes advice to eliminate smoking because, in individuals that smoke, drug effects may be:

    a. potentiated.

    *b. lessened.

    c. reach toxic levels.

    d. cancelled.

    Reference: p. 236

Cecil Landry, age 45, who is married and the sole support of his wife and 6 children, recently lost his job as an executive in the petroleum industry. He is seen by an out-patient clinic physician for complaints of irritability, agitation, and anxiety. The psychiatrist to whom he is referred diagnoses his condition as a situational anxiety and prescribes chlordiazepoxide (Librium) 10 mg 4 times a day.

4. The nurse explains to the patient that the chlordiazepoxide (Librium) prescribed for treatment of his anxiety is not likely to be extended beyond 4-5 months because:

    a. toxic effects will develop.

    b. coping skills will be lost.

    *c. physical dependence may occur.

    d. non-compliance is likely.

    Reference: p. 233

5. In teaching the patient about his prescribed medication of chlordiazepoxide (Librium), the nurse should explain that a common side-effects experienced in early stages of therapy is:

    a. memory impairment.

    *b. daytime drowsiness.

    c. urinary retention.

    d. vivid dreaming.

    Reference: p. 234

6. In his medication history, the patient taking chlordiazepoxide (Librium) reports he takes the following drugs. Of those listed, the one that prolongs the half-life of chlordiazepoxide leading to its cumulative effect is:

    *a. cimetidine (Tagamet)

    b. antacid (Maalox).

    c. ibuprofen (Advil).

    d. docusate sodium (Colace).

    Reference: p. 236

7. Three weeks after beginning therapy with chlordiazepoxide (Librium), the patient is admitted to the emergency department with symptoms of overdose (CNS depression, respiratory distress). The drug employed in cases of benzodiazepine overdose and the one the patient is likely to receive is:

    a. midazolam (Versed).

    b. prazepam (Centrax)

    *c. flumazenil (Romazicon).

    d. amphetamine sulfate.

    Reference: p. 238

8. Health teaching for the patient who is receiving midazolam (Versed) IM prior to a cardiac catheterization procedure would include informing the patient that:

*b. they may have some loss of memory for subsequent events.

c. swelling/burning at the site of injection is common.

d. salivation and retching is often experienced by patients.

Reference: p. 237

9. Patrice Humbolt, an 18 year old college freshman has recently ended her 2 year relationship with her high-school sweetheart. She presents at the student health center with complaints of generalized anxiety. In addition to referring Patrice to the counseling center, the nurse practitioner prescribes buspirone (BuSpar) 5 mg 3 times a day. In comparison to the benzodiazepines, buspirone (BuSpar) is unique in that it:

a. has a very rapid onset of action.

b. results in more adverse reactions

*c. does not interact with CNS depressants.

d. has a high potential for abuse.

Reference: p. 239

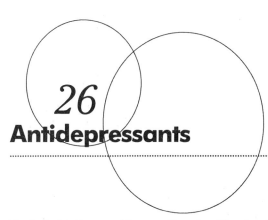

26
Antidepressants

Dr. Julia Merisco, a 40 year old university physiology professor sees a psychiatrist because of complaints of a prevailing loss of interest in pleasurable activities, excessive sleep, inability to concentrate, and a feeling that life is not worth living. The psychiatrist diagnoses her condition as endogenous depression and, in addition to psychotherapy, she prescribes imipramine (Tofranil) 50 mg 2 times a day.

1. The nurse explains to the patient that the antidepressant that the primary process through which the effects of imipramine (Tofranil) is mediated is:

   a. inhibiting the uptake of serotonin.

   b. inhibiting the uptake of an enzyme.

   c. stimulating the central nervous system..

   *d. blockade of biogenic amine uptake.

   Reference: p. 244

2. Following 4 weeks of effective therapy with imipramine (Tofranil) the patient says to the nurse, "When I get up quickly, I feel dizzy and faint and almost lose my balance." Health teaching by the nurse should be based on the probability that the patient is:

   a. drinking excessive caffeine.containing fluids.

   *b. suffering from orthostatic hypotension..

   c. getting too much of the prescribed drug.

   d. not getting enough aerobic exercise.

   Reference: p. 245

3. Drugs taken concurrently with imipramine (Tofranil) that may reduce its therapeutic effects are:

   a. urinary alkalinizers.

   *b. oral contraceptives.

   c. thyroid drugs.

   d. H₂ receptor antagonists.

   Reference: p. 247

4. In patients who are receiving antidepessants, the nurse needs to be particularly vigilant to the possibility of suicide when the patient:

   a. speaks slowly and in a monotone.

   b. is first starting drug therapy.

   c. is quizzed about suicidal ideation.

   *d. experiences lessened depression.

   Reference: p. 248

5. During the early stages of drug therapy with imipramine (Tofranil), the patient complains of excessive drowsiness. In addition to reassuring the patient that many of the side effects seen early in therapy diminish or disappear, which of the following of the nurse's suggestions would be most helpful to offset this effect?

   a. "Take a long nap in the middle of the day."

   b. "Drink one or two caffeine containing drinks."

   *c. "Request a once-a-day PM form of the drug."

   d. "Seek social stimulation and companionship."

   Reference: p. 246

6. A contraindication to the use of imipramine (Tofranil) is:

   a. history of dysmenorrhea.

   b. documentation of hypertension.

   c. history of peptic ulcer disease.

   *d. indication of breast-feeding.

   Reference: p. 248

7. In comparison to the tricyclic antidepessants, the tetracyclic antidepressant maprotiline (Ludiomil):

   a. is more delayed in onset and longer acting.

   b. is used to treat obsessive-compulsive disorder.

   *c. has fewer anti-cholinergic side effects.

   d. may be discontinued abruptly without any effects.

   Reference: pgs. 246—247

8. A typical antidepressants exhibiting selective inhibition of serotonin uptake in the brain and having comparatively fewer sedative and anticholinergic effects than do other antidepressants include all of the following except:

   a. fluoxetine (Prozac).

   b. paroxetine (Paxil).

   c. sertraline (Zoloft).

*d. tranylcypromine (Arnate).

Reference: p. 248

9. Pepper Morrison is being treated with an MAO inhibitor, isocarboxazid (Marplan), for chronic severe depression. Because of the danger of precipitating a hypertensive crisis, health teaching should include instructions to avoid foods containing:

a. vitamin C.

*b. tyramines.

c. purines.

d. licorice.

Reference: p. 251

10. Following the last dose of an MAO inhibitor, the patient should be warned to avoid all hazardous food and drugs for approximately:

a. one week.

*b. three weeks

c. two months.

d. four months.

Reference: p. 253

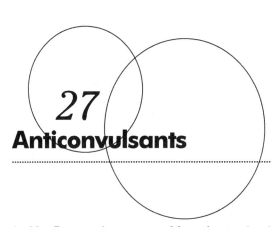

27
Anticonvulsants

1. Mr. Brown, is a year old patient who has been newly diagnosed with a seizure disorder for which he has been taking phenytoin (Dilantin). He says that lately he has not been getting good results from the Dilantin as he has begun to have some seizures. You tell Mr. Brown:

   a. "Your doctor will increase the dosage of your Dilantin, and if that doesn't help within the next few days, we can increase the dosage again."

   b. "It is to be expected that you continue to have seizures for a while after starting a new medication."

   c. "We may need to change the medication that you are taking quite frequently. "

   *d. "The dosage of Dilantin that you need may change if you are under stress."

   Reference: p. 255

2. An appropriate action for the neonatal nurse to take when caring for an infant born to a mother who is taking anticonvulsants is:

   *a. administration of vitamin K.

   b. administration of an anticonvulsant.

   c. administration of a sedative.

   d. institution of assisted ventilation.

   Reference: p. 257

3. In taking anticonvulsant medication, it is important that the patients understand that if the medication is discontinued,

   a. it must be replaced with another.

   *b. it must be gradually withdrawn.

   c. blood levels usually drop abruptly.

   d. it will be safe to drive.

   Reference: p. 255

4. Common adverse reactions to Dilantin include:

   a. renal and hepatic symptoms.

   b. CNS symptom of drowsiness

   c. paresthesias and decreased deep tendon reflexes.

   *d. skin rash and gum hyperplasia.

Reference: p. 259

5. During Mr. Brown's long-term therapy with Dilantin, he needs to be assessed for:

   a. CNS symptoms such as increased deep tendon reflexes.

   *b. early signs of blood dyscrasias.

   c. difficulty in urinating.

   d. hearing difficulties.

   Reference: p. 260

6. You should question the order if Dilantin is ordered for:

   a. Grand Mal seizures.

   b. Alcohol withdrawal syndrome.

   c. Trigeminal neuralgia.

   *d Petit Mal seizures.

   Reference: p. 259

7. You learn while talking to Mr. Brown that he knows very little about the hydantoin that he is taking. Your statements to him include all but:

   a. "Hydantoins react with many medications, so it is best not to take any over the counter medications unless your doctor instructs you to do so."

   b. "Good oral hygiene is very important."

   c. "Don't be alarmed if your urine turns pink."

   *d. "Avoid taking your medication with food."

   Reference: p. 260

8. A medication that is highly effective for Jacksonian seizures is:

   *a. Mephenytoin (Mesantoin).

   b. Hydantoin (Dilantin).

   c. Phenobarbital.

   d. Ethosuximide (Zarontin).

   Reference: p. 259

9. The principal indication for the use of Diazepam (Valium) is:

a. Petit Mal seizures.

b. Grand Mal seizures.

c. Jacksonian seizures.

*d. Status epilepticus.

Reference: p. 265

10. It is important to question the order if IV Diazepam is ordered for:

*a. Petit Mal seizures.

b. Grand Mal seizures.

c. Jacksonian seizures.

d. Absence seizures.

Reference: p. 265

11. A drug that is valuable as an adjunct to control absence or petit mal seizures is:

a. phenobarbital

b. Diazepam (Valium).

c. Ethosuximide (Zarontin).

*d. Acetazolamide (Diamox).

Reference: p. 265

12. Carbamazepine (Tegretol) may cause which of these adverse effects?

a. Hypertension

b. Dyspnea

c. Extrapyramidal symptoms

*d. Blood dyscrasias.

Reference: p. 267

13. Contraindications to the use of carbamazepine (Tegretol) include:

a. Lupus erythematosus

b. History of peptic ulcer disease

*c. History of bone marrow depression.

d. Glaucoma

Reference: p. 267

14. Patients taking Carbamazepine (Tegretol) should be sure to report to their physicians which of the following symptoms?

a. Drowsiness.

*b. Recurrent nosebleeds.

c. Urinary frequency

d. Diarrhea

Reference: p. 267

15. When administering magnesium sulfate, an important assesssment for the nurse to perform frequently is:

*a. Deep tendon reflexes.

b. Audiometry.

c. Liver palpation.

d. Inspection for petechiae.

Reference: p. 269

16. During administration of IV magnesium sulfate, which medication is kept on hand to administer intravenously as an antidote?

a. Procainamide.

b. Atropine.

c. Pronestyl.

*d. Calcium.

Reference: p. 270

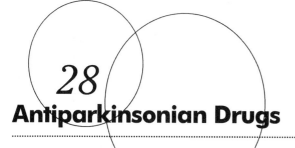

28
Antiparkinsonian Drugs

1. The symptoms of parkinsonism are caused by:
   a. Interruptions in cholinergic neural pathways.
   b. Excessive parasympathetic stimulation.
   c. Autonomic hypoactivity and decreased response in the peripheral system.
   *d. Low dopamine activity and high cholinergic action.
   Reference: p. 273

2. Because of her parkinsonism, your patient will have difficulty with:
   a. urinating, because the bladder muscle contracts only with difficulty.
   b. swallowing food or water.
   *c. reaching for a glass of water.
   d. sitting for any length of time.
   Reference: p. 273

3. The motor defect most responsive to treatment with levodopa is:
   a. Tremor.
   b. Rigidity.
   c. "Pill-rolling."
   *d. Akinesia.

   Reference: p. 274

4. In taking the medical history of a client who is to receive carbidopa/L-dopa (Sinemet) for Parkinsonism, the nurse should be especially alert to a history of:
   a. Hemolytic anemia.
   b. Hypertension.
   *c. Narrow angle-glaucoma.
   d. Myelitis.

   Reference: p. 275

5. The effects of L-dopa are potentiated by:
   a. chlorpromazine (Thorazine)

   b. phenytoin (Dilantin)
   c. reserpine (Serpasil)
   *d. propranolol (Inderal)
   Reference: p. 273

6. Before treatment with L-dopa is begun, it is important to assess your client for the presence of:
   *a. undiagnosed skin lesions.
   b. enlarged lymph glands.
   c. signs of bleeding.
   d. unequal pupillary response.
   Reference: p. 273

7. If adverse reactions to L-dopa are too great, a strategy is to combine the drug with another medication to allow smaller doses of L-dopa. One of the drugs used in this instance is:
   *a. benztropine (Cogentin).
   b. diazepam (Valium).
   c. procyclidine (Kemadrin).
   d. amantadine (Symmetrel).
   Reference: p. 277

9. The drug that may actually delay the progression of Parkinsonism is:
   a. bromocriptine (Arlodel).
   *b. selegiline (Eldepryl).
   c. procyclidine (Procyclid).
   d. amantadine (Symmetrel).
   Reference: p. 297

10. What medication in a patient's chart would lead you to question an order for trihexyphenidyl (Artane)?
    a. Antihistamine.
    b. Diuretic.
    c. Antihypertensive.
    *d. MAO inhibitor.
    Reference: p. 281

11. A side effect commonly found in patients taking anticholinergic/antihistaminergic agents include:

   a. hypertension.

   b. insomnia.

 *c. urinary hesitancy.

   d. diarrhea.

Reference: p. 280

29
Central Nervous System Stimulants

1. Albert Rush suffers from recurrent attacks of drowsiness and sleep during the daytime and falls asleep in the middle of conversations. He is diagnosed as having narcolepsy. As an adjunct to therapy, his physician is most likely to prescribe:

   a. caffeine (No Doz).

   b. doxapram (Dopram).

   *c. dextroamphetamine (Dexedrine).

   d. methamphetamine (Desoxyn).

   Reference: p. 286

2. The only appetite suppressant available without a prescription is:

   a. phenmetrazine Reference: reludin).

   b. mazindol (Sanorex).

   c. benzphetamine (Didrex).

   *d. phenylpropanolamine (Dexatrim).

   Reference: p. 288

3. Prescribed anorexiant drugs are used as an adjunct to the management of exogenous obesity. In relation to their use in obesity control, health teaching of the patient should include all of the following except:

   a. the importance of an exercise program.

   b. the need to continue caloric restriction.

   c. drugs will be prescribed for a limited time.

   *d. alleviating their fears about habituation.

   Reference: p. 289

4. Zacariah Bluecloud, who has insulin dependent diabetes mellitus, is involved in an obesity control program. His physician prescribed benzphetamine (Didex) 50 mg once a day at 10 am. In what way will the program affect his diabetic management?

   a. exercise will offset effects of hyperglycemia

   b. benzphetamine increases the need for insulin

   *c. weight loss may alter insulin needs.

   d. blood-glucose testing may be decreased.

   Reference: p. 287

5. Health teaching for patients who are taking amphetamine sulfate as part of an obesity management program should include to do all of the following except:

   *a. to stop the drug if mild hand tremors occur.

   b. to take the drug in the late afternoon.

   c. to increase caloric intake and exercise.

   d. to avoid excessive use of foods high in tyramine.

   Reference: p. 287

6. Luke Hammer, age 5, displays symptoms of inattention, impulsivity and hyperactivity and is diagnosed as having attention deficit disorder (ADD). A drug widely used as an adjunct to therapy for ADD and who's action is similar to amphetamine is:

   a. fenfluramine : ondimin).

   *b. methylphenidate (Ritalin).

   c. diethylpropion (Tenuate).

   d. phentermine (Ionamin).

   Reference: p. 290

7. Following general anesthesia to repair a hip fracture, William Tumba develops severe respiratory depression and is given doxapram (Dopram) to reverse it. The mechanism of action of this drug is mediated through:

   a. increasing the rate of metabolism of the anesthetic.

   *b. stimulation of peripheral carotid chemoreceptors.

   c. constriction of the cerebral blood vessels.

   d. mild stimulation of the cardiovascular system.

   Reference: p. 283

8. Following a cholecystectomy, Lorenzo Snick, a patient with chronic obstructive pulmonary disease, requires treatment with doxapram (Dopram). Planned nursing interventions for the patient would include all of the following except:

   a. assess arterial blood gases initially and every 30 minutes.

   b. mix the drug in normal saline or dextrose in water.

*c. plan to infuse the drug over a 24 hour period.

d. use an IV control pump to regulate the infusion rate.

Reference: p. 284

9. Robbie Eibbor occasionally develops a moderately severe headache. She has found that the use of an OTC analgesic containing caffeine to be more effective than one without it. In addition to the pain relief from the analgesic in the medication, the caffeine:

*a. causes stimulation of the CNS.

b. decreases skeletal muscle tone.

c. decreases neuronal firing.

d. slows respiratory and cardiac rate.

Reference: p. 285

III

Drugs Acting On The Cardiovascular System

30
Cardiovascular Physiology: A Review

1. A rapid heart rate is a potentially critical situation in patients with coronary atherosclerosis because of the reduced coronary perfusion secondary to:

   a. a shortened period of systole.

   *b. a shortened period of diastole.

   c. decreased peripheral resistence

   d. increased atrial emptying.

   Reference: p. 295

2. Autoregulation of coronary perfusion is known to be related to a number of factors. Coronary arteries dilate in response to all of the following *except:*

   a. increased H^+ ion levels.

   b. increased CO_2 levels

   c. increased potassium levels.

   *d. increased oxygen levels.

   Reference: p. 295

3. The area of the myocardium that undergoes the most rapid depolarization and, therefore, serves as the cardiac pacemaker is the:

   a. atrioventricular node.

   b. the bundle of His.

   *c. sinoatrial node.

   d. Purkinje fibers.

   Reference: p. 296

4. Cardiac function is directly affected by all of the following *except:*

   a. sympathetic nervous system.

   *b. the sensory cortex.

   c. serum electrolyte levels.

   d. decreased coronary blood flow.

   Reference: p. 296

5. The electrical activity of the heart is recorded graphically in the electrocardiogram (ECG). The part of the ECG tracing that indicates both ventricular depolarization and repolarization is the:

   a. the QRS interval

   b. the PR interval

   c. the T wave.

   *d. the QT interval

   Reference: p. 297

6. Delay in conduction of the myocardial electrical impulse at the AV node known as "heart block" is exhibited by:

   a. prolongation of the QT interval

   b. flattening of the T wave.

   *c. prolongation of the PR interval.

   d. shortening of the QRS complex.

   Reference: p. 297

7. An example of a drug induced change in the EKG is a flattened or inverted T wave secondary to:

   a. warfarin overdose.

   b. aspirin toxicity.

   c. allergy to cimetidine.

   *d. digitalis overdose.

   Reference: p. 297

8. The cardiac output in the normal resting adult of average size is:

   a. three liters per minute.

   *b. five liters per minute.

   c. seven liters per minute.

   d. nine liters per minute.

   Reference: p. 298

9. An important factor contributing to cardiac output is "preload" which describes the:

   a. Frank Starling Law of the Heart

   *b. stretch of myocardial fibers before contraction.

   c. tension a ventricle develops during systole.

   d. resistence to blood outflow from the ventricle.

   Reference: p. 298

10. High blood pressure and stenosis of the semilunar valves leads to:

    a. increased preload.

b. decreased afterload.

*c. increased afterload.

d. decreased preload.

Reference: p. 298

11. Intrinsic autoregulatory control factors that maintain local tissue blood flow by causing vasodilation include all of the following *except*:

a. nitric oxide.

b. lack of oxygen.

*c. endothelins.

d. increased metabolism.

Reference: p. 299

12. Humoral agents (hormones) that increase peripheral vascular resistence, thereby raising the blood pressure include all of the following *except*:

*a. bradykinin.

b. catecholamines.

c. angiotensin II.

d. vasopressin.

Reference: p. 299

13. By definition, the mean arterial pressure is equal to the:

a. lowest pressure in the arteries just before systole.

*b. diastolic pressure plus one-third of the pulse pressure.

c. difference between systolic and diastolic pressure.

d. pressure occurring at the peak of ventricular contraction.

Reference: p. 299

14. Increased levels of angiotensin II produces increased blood pressure through all of the following mechanisms *except*:

a. increasing aldosterone production.

b. direct stimulation of the vascular muscle.

c. causing arteriole vasoconstriction.

*d. stimulation of the baroreceptors.

Reference: p. 200

31
Cardiotonic Drugs

....

1. Drugs that have a positive inotropic action on the heart muscle, thus increasing the force of contraction and improving its functional ability include all of the following *except:*

   a. deslanoside (Cedilanid-D)

   b. digitoxin (Crystodigin)

   c. amrinone (Inocor).

   *d. lidocaine (LidoPen).

   Reference: pgs. 302—306

2. The purposes of initiating drug therapy with digitalis by administration of high ("loading") doses include all of the following *except:*

   a. to achieve high serum levels quickly.

   b. to produce an immediate therapeutic effect.

   *c. to increase its rate of metabolism.

   d. to saturate the available receptor sites.

   Reference: p. 302

3. Jana Titan is receiving large doses of digoxin for the purpose of rapid digitalization to relieve symptoms of acute congestive heart failure. The nurse is aware of the increased potential for digitalis toxicity if the patient has:

   a. simple constipation.

   b. a high serum osmolality.

   c. low hemoglobin level.

   *d. an increased creatinine level.

   Reference: p. 304

4. Increased serum levels of digitalis glycosides, therefore the possibility of digitalis toxicity, are associated with the use of all of the following *except:*

   *a. cimetidine

   b. quinidine.

   c. verapamil.

   d. nifedipine.

   Reference: p. 304

5. Xaviar Shalom is taking a digoxin (Lanoxin) 0. 125 mg, and a diuretic, furosemide (Lasix) 80 mg, daily for treatment of his congestive heart failure. In response to the patient's inquiry about what to do if he misses a dose of digoxin, the nurse would tell the patient to:

   a. take 2 doses of the drug the next day.

   b. report this oversight to his physician.

   *c. take the prescribed dose daily as usual.

   d. skip his next dose of the prescribed diuretic.

   Reference: p. 305

6. Health teaching for the patient taking digitalis includes instructing the individual to report signs and symptoms of toxicity. These include all of the following *except:*

   a. pulse rate below 60 per minute.

   b. diarrhea, nausea, vomiting.

   c. blurred vision, halo vision, diplopia.

   *d. muscle aching and joint stiffness.

   Reference: p. 305

7. Health teaching for the patient receiving digitalis and diuretics should include instructions to increase dietary intake of:

   *a. potassium-rich foods.

   b. foods high in soluble fiber.

   c. foods high in vitamin K.

   d. iron rich animal protein.

   Reference: p. 305

8. Miller Farkleberry is admitted to the acute care in-patient unit for treatment of life-threatening digoxin intoxication. The drug the nurse would expect to be administered to reverse the effects of the digitalis is:

   a. milrinone (Primacor).

   *b. digoxine immune fab (Digibind).

   c. quinidine (Cardioquin).

   d. bretylium (Bretylol).

   Reference: p. 306

9. The nurse should closely observe the patient who is taking amrinone (Inocor) for:

   a. elevated white blood counts.

   *b. arrhythmias.

   c. high blood pressure.

   d. seizures.

   Reference: p. 306

10. Which of the following solutions should be used by the nurse in preparing a prescribed maintenance infusion of amrinone (Inocor)?

    a. lactated Ringer's solution

    b. 5% dextrose in water

    *c. normal saline

    d. 5% dextrose in 0. 45 saline

    Reference: p. 307

32
Antiarrthymic Drugs

1. Patients taking quinidine (Quinaglute) should be advised to consume limited quantities of caffeine and alcohol, and to smoke in moderation because all of these contain substances that:

   a. increase liver enzyme activity.

   *b. alter the irritability of the heart.

   c. displace receptor binding sites.

   d. increase kidney excretion.

   Reference: p. 311

2. The nurse should inform the patient beginning quinidine therapy that a common early side effect (usually temporary) is:

   *a. diarrhea.

   b. impaired hearing.

   c. fine tremors.

   d. urticaria.

   Reference: p. 311

3. Electrocardiographic evidence of cardiotoxicity in patients receiving quinidine include all of the following *except*:

   a. widening of the QRS complex

   *b. peaked (tented) T waves.

   c. ventricular extrasystoles.

   d. abolition of P waves.

   Reference: p. 311

4. To decrease the risk of drug toxicity, health teaching of patients receiving quinidine should include instructions to avoid the consumption of large amounts of:

   a. potassium-rich foods.

   *b. citrus fruits.

   c. foods high in calcium.

   d. salty foods.

   Reference: p. 311

5. Following the correction of a ventricular arrhythmia, a patient is placed on maintenance therapy of sustained release procainamide (Procan SR) 250 mg every 6 hours. A serious adverse effect for which the nurse should plan to monitor the patient is:

   a. hypertension.

   *b. agranulocytosis.

   c. severe headache.

   d. hypoglycemia.

   Reference: p. 312

6. Houston Artmin's physician has prescribed disopyramide (Norpace) to prevent recurrent episodes of ventricular tachycardia. Nursing intervention would include the identification of the nursing diagnoses of:

   a. High risk for urge incontinence.

   *b. High risk for urinary retention.

   c. High risk for fluid volume deficit.

   d. High risk for injury.

   Reference: p. 313

7. An antiarrthymic used in the abolish acute ventricular arrhythmias resulting from myocardial infarction, cardiac manipulation, and digitalis intoxication is:

   a. phenytoin (Dilantin) IV.

   *b. lidocaine IV.

   c. quinidine IV

   d. propranalol IV

   Reference: p. 315

8. A patient with frequent PVCs is given an IV bolus of lidocaine 50 mg and then receives a continuous IV infusion of the drug over a period of several hours. The nurse expects the IV infusion rate to be adjusted to maintain a blood serum level at:

   *a. 2-5 mcg/ml.

   b. 5-8 mcg/ml.

   c. 8-11 mcg/ml.

   d. 11-14 mcg/ml.

   Reference: p. 315

66

9. Eldridge Blitzman's physician has prescribed tocainide (Tonocard) 400 mg, PO, every 8 hours, for the treatment of premature ventricular contractions. A nursing diagnosis essential to planning nursing interventions is:

a. High risk for activity intolerance

b. High risk for constipation

*c. High risk for injury

d. High risk for altered nutrition: More than body requirements

Reference: p. 316

10. A patient with a supraventricular tachycardia is admitted to a clinical unit for continuous EKG and blood pressure monitoring and is given verapamil 5 mg by IV push. If the arrhythmia is not terminated, the nurse should expect that the next dose may be administered within:

a. 15 minutes.

*b. 30 minutes.

c. 45 minutes.

d. 60 minutes.

Reference: p. 325

11. A patient is being treated with phenytoin (Dilantin) IV for an arrhythmia resulting from digitalis toxicity. A drug the nurse would have available for administration in the event that bradycardia or a heart block develops is:

*a. atropine.

b. captopril.

c. amyl nitrate.

d. calcium gluconate.

Reference: p. 325

12. The physician prescribe flecainide (Tambocor) 150 mg every 12 hours for the treatment of a patient with a ventricular arrhythmia. Health teaching by the nurse should include instructing the patient to report:

a. nausea, mild headache.

b. lightheadedness, minor visual changes.

c. constipation, feelings of fullness.

*d. rapid weight gain, shortness of breath.

Reference: p. 319

13. April Knox, 45 years old, is seen at an outpatient clinic for persistent tachycardia. The physician identifies the probable cause as thyrotoxicosis and to control her rapid heart rate is likely to prescribe:

a. propafenone.

*b. propranolol.

c. bretylium.

d. lidocaine.

Reference: p. 321

14. The physician prescribes amiodarone (Cordarone) 400 mg two times a day for a patient. Which of the following conditions in the patient's health history would alert the nurse to a contraindication for its use?

a. COPD

b. diabetes mellitus

c. hypertension

*d. sinus bradycardia

Reference: p. 323

15. The expected electrocardiogram (EKG) changes that occur from the effects of amiodarone (Cordarone) is:

a. decreased QT interval

*b. increased PR interval

c. inversion of the T wave

d. abolished P wave

Reference: p. 323

33
Antihypertensive Drugs

Dudley Buford is 62 years old, slightly overweight, and the president of a small university. He is referred for treatment to the local Veteran's Administration Blood Pressure Clinic because of a sustained blood pressure elevation averaging 160/100. The physician prescribes atenolol (Tenormin) 50 mg daily and hydrochlorothiazide (HCTZ) 25 mg daily and refers him to the clinic nurse for counseling.

1. Health teaching for patients with hypertension should include teaching them about nonpharmacological measures known to enhance its control. These include all of the following except:

   *a. limiting the amount of water intake.

   b. weight loss to achieve ideal body weight.

   c. increasing aerobic exercise as tolerated.

   d. learning to manage stressful situations.

   Reference: p. 327

Because Dr. Buford's blood pressure remains elevated with the combination atenolol and hydrochlorothiazide therapy, the physician adds captopril (Capoten) 25 mg three times a day to his drug regimen.

2. Captopril (Capoten) is an antihypertensive agent that is classified as:

   a. a sympathetic ganglionic blocker.

   *b. an angiotensin-converting enzyme inhibitor.

   c. an alpha-adrenergic nerve blocker.

   d. a direct acting peripheral vasodilator.

   Reference: p. 331

3. Patients taking captopril should be instructed to maintain the same salt intake as prior to initiating therapy to decrease the risk of:

   a. severe dehydration.

   b. congestive heart failure.

   *c. a precipitous decrease in BP.

   d. polyuria and proteinuria.

   Reference: p. 334

4. To enhance absorption of captopril, the patient should be instructed to take the medication:

   a. with milk. or a snack.

   b. during or right after meals.

   c. with citrus fruit juice.

   *d. an hour before meals with water.

   Reference: p. 334

5. All of the following factors are likely to contribute to a patient's noncompliance to antihypertensive therapy except:

   a. lack of symptoms of the disease.

   b. troublesome drug side-effects.

   *c. involvement in self-monitoring of BP.

   d. need for continued long-term therapy.

   Reference: pgs. 327—348

6. Sexual dysfunction, a particularly troublesome potential side effect of antihypertensive therapy, is most often associated with:

   a. diuretics.

   b. direct-acting vasodilators.

   c. ACE inhibitors.

   *d. alpha$_1$ andrenergic blocking agents.

   Reference: p. 334

7. Patients in which prazosin (Minipress) therapy is being initiated should be cautioned that it may cause a "first dose effect" of:

   a. urinary retention.

   b. explosive diarrhea.

   *c. severe postural hypotension.

   d. urinary frequency.

   Reference: p. 335

8. A physician prescribes prazosin (Minipress) l mg daily and hydrochlorthiazide 25 mg daily for a patient with moderate hypertension. In the initial stages of therapy with prazosin, patient instructions should emphasize:

   *a. changing positions slowly (supine to standing).

   b. taking the medication with a snack or meals.

68

c. increasing the intake of potassium rich foods.

d. limiting fluid intake to 1500 ml a day.

Reference: p. 335

9. A patient's physician has prescribed clonidine (Catapres) and a diuretic for the treatment of moderate hypertension. Health teaching by the nurse should include informing the patient that:

a. effects of the drug will increase over time.

*b. sensitivity to alcohol may be increased.

c. they may experience episodes of insomnia.

d. their appetite is likely to be increased.

Reference: p. 337

10. For management of a moderate form of hypertension, a p.340physician prescribes hydralazine (Apresoline) for a patient. Hydralazine is classified as a:

a. central alpha2 adrenergic agonist.

b. calcium channel blocker.

c. alpha1 adrenergic blocking agent.

*d. vascular smooth muscle relaxant.

Reference: p. 340

11. A drug that may be used to alleviate the symptoms of hydralazine-p.341 induced peripheral neuritis is:

a. vitamin C.

b. vitamin B12.

*c. pyridoxine.

d. vitamin A.

Reference: p. 341

12. Nursing interventions for patients receiving methyldopa should include instructions to report the following to their physician immediately:

a. a feeling of sedation.

b. dry mouth and nasal stuffiness.

*c. involuntary movements.

d. increased appetite and weight gain.

Reference: p. 338

13. A patient with difficult to control hypertension is receiving a combination of minoxidil (Loniten), a diuretic, and a beta-blocking agent. Health teaching should include informing the patient that a common side effect of minoxidil is:

a. hyperactivity.

b. drowsiness.

*c. hypertrichosis.

d. depression.

Reference: p. 341

14. A patient is admitted to the critical care unit because of severe hypertension (blood pressure ranges between 182/120 and 200/160 mm Hg). The physician prescribes nitroprusside (Nipride) IV at the rate of 3 mcg/kg/minute. The mechanism of action of nitroprusside is:

a. slowed heart rate and decreased vascular resistence.

*b. direct relaxation of arteriolar and venule smooth muscle

c. selective blockage of alpha1 receptor sites.

d. activation of presynaptic adrenergic alpha2 receptors.

Reference: p. 345

15. In patients being treated with intravenous nitroprusside, nursing interventions include frequent monitoring of the blood pressure and adjusting the infusion rate to achieve the desired response. The systolic blood pressure should not be allowed to fall below:

*a. 70 mm Hg.

b. 80 mm Hg.

c. 90 mm Hg.

d. 100 mm Hg.

Reference: p. 346

16. All of the following are important nursing considerations related to the preparation and administration of nitroprusside intravenous solutions *except:*

a. use the solutions within 4 hours of preparation.

b. cover the infusion container with an opaque material.

*c. discard solutions that have a faint brownish tinge.

d. do not add other drugs to the infusion solution.

Reference: p. 346

17. In patients receiving nitroprusside therapy continuing beyond 2—3 days, it is important to determine the the blood serum level of:

a. creatinine.

*b. thiocyanate.

c. renin.

d. sodium nitrate.

Reference: p. 346

34
Antianginals

1. An important goal in the treatment of your patient's angina is to increase the myocardial blood flow. It is also important to achieve:

   a. dilation of the coronary artery.

   b. selective vascular dilation.

   c. increased venous return to the heart.

   *d. reduction of the workload of the heart.

   Reference: p. 349

2. Beta Blockers are also helpful in the treatment of angina. Indications for the use of beta blockers include all except:

   a. angina during exertion

   b. tachyarrhythmias

   *c. severe attacks of angina when at rest.

   d. moderate hypertension.

   Reference: p. 357

3. In Mr. CQ's case, the physician has decided to use nitroglycerine gr 1/150 sublingually. When you teach him about his medication, you include all of these statements except:

   a. "You can take one of these tablets under your tongue if you are in a situation so stressful that it might cause an attack of angina."

   b. "Take up to three tablets a 5 minute intervals, but if your pain is not relieved, go to a hospital."

   *c. "If you notice that the pill is not working as well as it has been, increase the dosage to two pills."

   d. "Don't drink at the same time that you take these tablets."

   Reference: p. 355

4. Mr. CQ complains that the nitroglycerine gives him a headache. You advise him to:

   *a. lie down for about 30 minutes to see if the headache will subside during that time.

   b. eat a small amount of food before taking the tablet to prevent this side effect.

   c. take the nitroglycerine with aspirin to prevent the headache.

   d. swallow the pill to slow absorption and prevent the headache.

   Reference: p. 355

5. Mr. CQ is going on a trip and plans to put his nitroglycerine in a small cardboard box which is easily stored. You tell him:

   a. "You can take a topical nitroglycerine to relieve any acute attacks."

   *b. "Store the drug only in the original container."

   c. "Travel may increase your symptoms, so pack extra pills in a separate container to keep in your glove compartment."

   d. "Keep the pills in your inside shirt pocket, where it can stay warm and dissolve more readily."

   Reference: p. 351

6. The physician is considering the use of verapamil (Calan) in Mr. CQ's medication regime. In taking his history and performing a physical assessment, you are hesitant to give the drug when you note in his history:

   a. open-angle glaucoma.

   b. peptic ulcer and bleeding.

   *c. hypotension and bradycardia.

   d. hypertension and tachyarrhythmias.

   Reference: p. 353

7. During the initial stages of therapy with a calcium-channel blocker, you assess your patient carefully for problems with the medication. The assessments include all except:

   a. frequent blood pressure checks for hypotensive episodes.

   b. frequent ECGs to detect any bradycardia.

   c. pulmonary assessments to detect cardiac failure.

   *d. Blood studies to detect any hemolytic effects.

   Reference: p. 356

8. After her myocardial infarction, your patient, Ms.Smith, is taking nadolol (Corgard) to treat her angina. What is the action of this drug that would benefit Ms.Smith?

 a. Blockage of the flow of calcium ions into the smooth muscle tissue within the vascular system.

 b. Reduction of the excitability of the conductive tissue within the SA and AV nodes.

 *c. Blockage of the beta receptors within the smooth muscle tissue of the vascular system.

 d. It acts as a "direct vasodilator," and affects only the coronary artery.

 Reference: p. 357

9. The physician also has prescribed nitroglycerine patches for Ms.Smith. The rationale behind the addition of the patch to her regime is that it will:

 a. potentiate the action of Corgard.

 b. decrease the automaticity of the ventricular tissues.

 c. decrease myocardial oxygen consumption.

 *d. decrease peripheral resistance.

 Reference: p. 349

10. Yet another drug, dipyridamole (Persantine) 75 mg po qid, is added to Ms. Smith's regime. Dipyridamole, which is often used after a myocardial infarction, is prescribed because of it's action best described as:

 *a. coronary vasodilation and inhibitor of platelet aggregation.

 b. nonselective beta blockade and inhibitor of cardiac action.

 c. peripheral vascular dilator and hypotensive agent.

 d. vascular smooth muscle relaxant and slow channel blocker.

 Reference: p. 357

11. The rationale behind the physician's selection of dipyridamole is that:

 a. Dipyridamole may reduce the inflammatory effects of myocardial ischemia.

 b. Arrhythmias can be stabilized through the use of dipyridamole.

 c. The drug could reduce hyperlipidemia

 *d. Another MI may be prevented by the use of this drug.

 Reference: p. 357

12. Patients taking Cyclandelate (Cyclospasmol) need to be watched for:

 a. anorexia, dry mouth

 *b. bleeding tendencies.

 c. lethargy, depression.

 d. urticaria.

 Reference: p. 359

13. A peripheral vasodilator used to provide symptomatic relief of signs of mental decline in the elderly is:

 a. Cyclandelate (Cyclan).

 b. Isoxsuprine (Vasodilan).

 *c. Ergoloid mesylate (Hydergine).

 d. Isoxsuprine (Vasodilan).

 Reference: p. 359

14. Your elderly patient is taking papaveine (Pavabid) to relieve symptoms of cerebral ischemia. Which effect of the peripheral vasodilator would pose a hazard to your elderly patient?

 *a. Significant hypotension occurs with the administration of peripheral vasodilators.

 b. The peripheral vasodilators do not relieve the ischemia of vascular disease to any great extent.

 c. Peripheral vasodilators do not increase the blood flow distal to an occlusion.

 d. Blood flow is increased primarily to non-ischemic areas by peripheral vasodilators.

 Reference: pgs. 358—359

35
Prophylaxis of Atherosclerosis: Hypolipemic Drugs

1. Risk factors for the development of atherosclerosis include all of the following except:

   a. elevated plasma levels of LDL.

   b. consumption of saturated animal fat.

   *c. increased plasma levels of HDL.

   d. high blood pressure.

   Reference: p. 361

2. Nursing assessment of patient's taking bile acid sequestering resins should include the close monitoring of:

   *a. bleeding time

   b. thrombocyte count

   c. white blood count

   d. serum calcium

   Reference: p. 362

3. Nursing assessment of the patient taking bile acid sequestering resins should include evaluations for nutritional deficiencies related to:

   a. essential fatty acids.

   b. cholesterol.

   c. water-soluble vitamins.

   *d. fat-soluble vitamins.

   Reference: p. 362

4. Patients who are taking colestipol (Colestid) should be taught to take the drug:

   a. on an empty stomach with water.

   b. with an antacid.

   *c. mixed with liquid food or water.

   d. at bedtime with a snack.

   Reference: p. 363

5. Education for the patient taking bile acid sequestering resins should include instructions to ingest other prescribed oral medications:

   *a. 1 hour before or 4 hours after the resin.

   b. with the resin previously dissolved in water.

   c. with an antacid and the resin.

   d. within twenty minutes of resin intake.

   Reference: p. 363

6. To minimize a common side-effect associated with cholestyramine (Questran) therapy, nursing intervention should include instructions to prevent:

   a. nausea.

   *b. constipation.

   c. decreased appetite.

   d. diarrhea.

   References: p. 363

7. In patients taking antilipemic drugs, as clofibrate (Astromid-S), nursing interventions should emphasize the need:

   *a. to adhere to a low-cholesterol diet.

   b. to avoid exposure to the sun.

   c. to avoid OTC aspirin products.

   d. for a yearly lipid profile.

   Reference: p. 365

8. Which of the following laboratory test results should the nurse expect to monitor periodically in the patient taking gemfibrozil (Lopid)?

   a. bleeding time

   *b. liver function tests

   c. magnesium levels

   d. thyroid hormone levels

   Reference: p. 366

9. Health teaching for the patient taking gemfibrozil (Lopid) would include informing the patient that a common side effect associated with therapy is:

   a. back pain, myalgia, muscle cramping.

   b. flatulence, belching, anorexia.

   c. rash, pruritus, dry skin.

   *d. abdominal pain, diarrhea, nausea.

   Reference: p. 366

10. A physician prescribes lovastatin (Mevacor) 20 mg once daily for a patient with hypercholesterolemia

that has failed to respond to non-pharmacologic interventions. The nurse should instruct the patient to take the medication:

a. on awakening.

b. with breakfast.

c. with the noon meal.

*d. in the evening.

Reference: p. 368

11. A patient's physician has prescribed nicotinic acid (Niacin) as adjunctive therapy for hyperlipidemia. To help reduce the flushing associated with its use, the nurse instructs the patient to:

a. take the drug with a large glass of cold water.

b. drink a hot beverage and then take the drug.

c. chew the tablets completely before swallowing.

*d. take 325 mg of aspirin 30 minutes before taking the drug.

Reference: p. 369

36
Antianemic Drugs

1. The symptoms of anemia are caused by:
   a. reduced levels of folic acid.
   b. inhibition of the absorption of iron from the GI tract.
   *c. inadequate tissue oxygenation.
   d. transient neurologic disability.
   Reference: p. 371

2. Red cells are formed in the:
   a. spleen.
   *b. bone marrow.
   c. liver
   d. gastric epithelium
   Reference: p. 371

3. The substances required for the formation of red blood cells include all except:
   a. iron
   b. folic acid
   c. vitamin B12
   d. nicotinic acid
   Reference: p. 371

4. Deficiency anemias are referred to as:
   a. aplastic
   b. hemolytic
   c. hypochromic
   d. megaloblastic
   Reference: p. 371

5. Anemias that are caused by insufficient levels of folic acid or B12 are known as:
   a. aplastic
   b. hemolytic
   c. hypochromic
   d. hyperchromic
   Reference: p. 371

6. Anemias that are the result of drug toxicity are termed:
   a. aplastic
   b. microcytic
   c. hypochromic
   d. megaloblastic
   Reference: p. 371

7. To enchance absorption, your patient taking an oral iron preparation needs to be instructed to take the medication with:
   a. milk
   b. maalox
   c. toast or crackers
   d. orange juice
   Reference: p. 373

8. Before you give Iron Dextran IM to your patient for the first time, it is important that you:
   a. check H&P for a history of phlebitis.
   b. order a cratinine level to varify normal renal function.
   c. assess the potassium levels to be sure hypokalemia is not a problem.
   d. give 1/2 cc to test for an allergic reaction.
   Reference: p. 373

9. An indication for the use of IV Iron Dextran is:
   a. poor oral absorption.
   b. Hb below 9 gm/dl.
   c. uncontrolled bleeding.
   d. increased muscle mass.
   Reference: p. 373

10. In giving Iron Dextran intramuscularly, it is important to use this route:
    a. subcutaneous with a 1/2" needle.
    b. deep IM into the deltoid with a 2"–3" needle.
    c. into the gluteus maximus with a 1"–1 1/2" needle.
    d. z-track with a 2"–3" needle into the gluteus maximus.
    Reference: p. 374

11. The result of folic acid and vitamin B_{12} deficiency is:

   *a. inhibition of normal cell division.

   b. inhibition of hemoglobin synthesis.

   c. inhibition of red blood cell production.

   d. bone marrow depression.

   Reference: p. 374

12. Symptoms that your patient exhibits that are characteristic of pernicious anemia would be:

   a. A sore tongue and tingling hands.

   b. loose blck, tarry stools

   c. bradycardia and fatigue.

   d. unexplained weight gain.

   Reference: p. 375

13. Instructions for your patient taking injection of cyanocobalamin would include all except:

   a. "Response to the injections may take a number of weeks, as your recovery may be slow."

   b. "The neurologic symptoms will be relieved by the injections, and further damage will be prevented."

   c. "It is important to take the shots regularly to prevent progressive nerve damage."

   d. "If you become ill, you need to have the dosage of the medication increased."

   Reference: pgs. 375—376

14. The action of Folic Acid results in:

   a. the release of elemental iron

   b. the activation of coenzymes necessary for the synthesis of red blood cells.

   c. facilitation of the absorption of cyanocobalamin.

   d. the production of red blood cells and platelets.

   Reference: p. 376

15. Indications for the use of Folic Acid include:

   a. simple pernicious anemia.

   b. aplastic anemia caused by drug usage.

   c. normocytic anemias seen in malnutrition.

   d. megaloblastic anemias seen in alcoholism.

   Reference: p. 376

16. Your education for your patient who is taking Folic Acid includes this statement:

   a. "Salmon is high in Folic Acid."

   b. "Be sure to eat extra fruit and green vegetables every day."

   c. "Supplement your diet with Folic Acid if you notice symptoms of fatigue and lethargy returning."

   d. "You may not notice any improvement for several weeks after you state your supplements."

   Reference: p. 377

17. The metabolite of Folic Acid used to minimize the cellular toxicity that results from the use of methotrexate is:

   a. Ferrous fumarate (Feostat).

   b. Polysaccharide-Iron Complex (Nu-iron).

   c. Leucovorin (Wellcovorin).

   d. Ferrous Gluconate (Fergon).

   Reference: p. 377

37
Anticoagulants/Thrombolytic/Hemostatic

1. The two pathways of clot formation are called:
   a. thrombolytic and hemostatic
   b. anticoagulant and antithrombic
   *c. intrinsic and extrinsic
   d. coagulant and fibrinogenic
   Reference: p. 378

2. Drugs that *prevent* the formation of new clots are called:
   *a. anticoagulants.
   b. thrombolytics.
   c. hemostatics.
   d. antihemorrhagics.
   Reference: p. 378

3. Drugs that *enhance* the formation of new clots are called:
   a. anticoagulants.
   b. thrombolytics.
   *c. hemostatics.
   d. antihemorrhagics.
   Reference: p. 378

4. Heparin is used for all of the following *except*:
   a. as an anticoagulant in blood transfusion.
   b. prevention of cerebral thrombosis in evolving stroke.
   c. treatment of DIC
   *d. prophylaxis in patients with prosthetic valves.
   Reference: p. 379

5. You know that the heparin dosage is adequate when the patient's PTT partial thromboplastin time) is:
   a. 1/3 to 1/2 of the control value.
   b. equal to the control value.
   *c. 1 1/2 to 2 times the control value.
   d. 2 to 2 1/2 times the control value.
   Reference: p. 379

6. Your patient who is taking heparin complains of a headache and asks for aspirin to ease his discomfort. Your most appropriate action is to:
   a. after clarification from the physician, give aspirin no more frequently than every 6 hours for headache.
   b. give ibuprofen with food or milk.
   c. reassure the patient that this reaction is not unusual and will resolve itself.
   *d. contact the physician for an order for acetaminophen.
   Reference: p. 381

7. In case of heparin overdosage, the heparin antagonist that must be administered is:
   a. injectable vitamin K.
   *b. Protamine Sulfate.
   c. Factors IX, I, and II
   d. Dicumoral
   Reference: p. 381

8. In giving parenteral heparin, the correct nursing action is to:
   a. give deep IM in gluteal tissue to minimize irritation.
   b. massage the area after administration to enhance absorption.
   c. aspirate before injecting the heparin.
   *d. give subcutaneously, using a Z track technique.
   Reference: p. 381

9. Your patient has been placed on long term heparin therapy. Your teaching will include all statements except:
   a. "Use acetaminophen in preference to ibuprofen."
   b. "Notify your practitioner if you notice unusual bruising or back pain."
   *c. "Be sure to take aspirin or ibuprofen with food."
   d. "Tell every health care provider who takes care of you that you are taking heparin. "
   Reference: p. 381

10. The longest acting anticoagulant is:
    a. heparin
    b. warfarin
    *c. dicumarol
    d. anisindione
    Reference: p. 383

11. Which patient is most likely to be placed on cou-
    madin therapy?
    a. The newly admitted patient who has an un-
       confirmed diagnosis of cerebrovascular
       hemorrhage.
    *b. The patient with a newly placed prosthetic
       valve.
    c. The diabetic patient with an MI.
    d. The patient with subacute bacterial endocarditis.

    Reference: p. 383

12. Which statement would be included in your
    teaching for the patient on coumadin?
    *a. "Don't change the amounts of green, leafy vege-
       tables that you eat daily."
    b. "If you forget a dose, double your next dose."
    c. "It is not necessary to ask us about any over the
       counter drugs that you may need to take."
    d. "Daily labs are important while you are on main-
       tenance therapy."

    Reference: p. 384

13. Your diabetic patient, Mr. Jones, has been well
    maintained on acetohexamide (Dymelor) for a
    number of years. What change might you see
    when he is started on Dicumarol?
    *a. A decrease in blood sugar, as Dicumarol po-
       tentiates the action of Dymelor.
    b. Poor response to the Dicumarol, as Dymelor
       blocks the action of this drug.
    c. An increase in blood sugar, as Dicumarol
       blocks the action of Dymelor.
    d. An exaggerated response to the Dicumarol, as
       Dymelor potentiates the action of Dicumarol.

    Reference: p. 384

14. The medication used as an antidote for over-
    dosage of *oral* anticoagulant drugs is:
    a. heparin.
    b. protamine
    *c. vitamin K.
    d. vitamin E.
    Reference: p. 385

15. The drug of choice for the treatment of intermit-
    tent claudication is:
    a. Dicumarol.
    b. Coumadin.
    c. heparin.
    *d. Trental.
    Reference: p. 386

16. After a myocardial infarction, the timing of throm-
    bolysis is crucial. Therapy should begin how soon
    after the onset of symptoms?
    *a. 4 hours.
    b. 8 hours.
    c. 14 hours.
    d. 48 hours.
    Reference: p. 387

17. The drug used to treat an overdose of streptoki-
    nase is:
    a. phytonadione (Aquamephyton).
    b. heparin.
    c. protamine sulfate.
    *d. aminocaproic acid (Amicar).
    Reference: p. 389

18. Ms. O. experiences a severe nosebleed during her
    therapy with Streptokinase. Your response
    should be to:
    a. discontinue her infusion.
    b. prepare to administer whole blood.
    *c. apply pressure, draw PTT.
    d. prepare to give a hemostatic.
    Reference: p. 389

19. During streptokinase therapy, appropriate nursing
    actions include:
    *a. Maintain the patient on bedrest.
    b. Frequent monitoring of PTT.
    c. Encouragement and assistance in frequent
       turning and position changes.
    d. Frequent arterial punctures for ABGs.
    Reference: p. 289

20. When administering Streptokinase, the nurse's
    actions include,
    a. mixing with sterile water.
    b. shake well to mix.
    *c. further dilution with 100 ml of solution,
    d. inject IV over 5 min.
    Reference: p. 388

21. The drug of choice that is used to restore patency to IV catheters is:

    a. alteplase (Activase).

    b. streptokinase (Kabikinase).

    c. anistreplase (Eminase).

    *d. urokinase (Abbokinase).

    Reference: p. 388

22. Contraindications to the administration of Human Antihemophilic factors include:

    a. severe hemorrhage.

    b. the presence of viral hepatitis.

    *c. inhibitors to factor VIII.

    d. deficiency of factor VIII.

    Reference: p. 391

NOTES

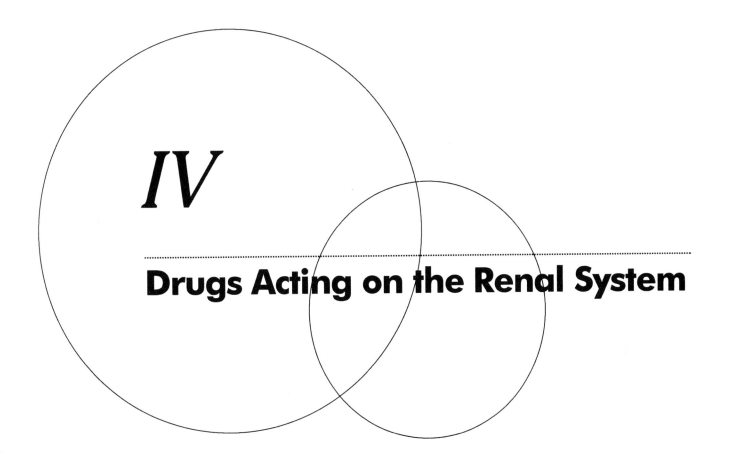

IV

Drugs Acting on the Renal System

38
Renal

1. The basic unit of the kidney that performs most of the work of the kidney is the:

  a. medulla.

  *b. nephron.

  c. Bowman's capsule.

  d. calyx

  Reference p. 401

2. The response of the juxtaglomerular cells to decreased renal perfusion, hypotension or hyperkalemia is the secretion of:

  a. MSH.

  b. aldosterone.

  c. ACTH.

  *d. renin.

  Reference: p. 402

3. The kidneys receive what percentage of the cardiac output in the adult at rest?

  a. 10%-15%

  *b. 20%-25%

  c. 30%-35%

  d. 40%-45%

  Reference: p. 402

4. The amount of urine produced by the kidneys is *ultimately* dependent upon the:

  a. colloidal osmotic pressures within the Bowman's capsule.

  b. glomerular capillary hydrostatic pressure.

  *c. work of the heart and the resulting output.

  d. a stable blood pressure within 20-30 mm of normal.

  Reference: p. 403

5. The percentage of plasma reabsorbed in a 24 hour period totals about:

  a. 25%

  b. 56%

  *c. 70%

d. 99%

  Reference: p. 403

6. The average amount of urine produced per day is:

  a. 1/2 to one liter.

  *b. between 1 1/2 to 2 liters.

  c. between 2 1/2 to 3 liters.

  d. about 3 1/2 liters.

  Reference p. 403

7. Reabsorption and secretion of substances takes place in the:

  a. Bowman's capsule.

  *b. renal tubules.

  c. medullary pyramid.

  d. renal cortex.

  Reference: p. 303

8. Renal failure may interfere with the excretion of some therapeutic agents and the strategy most helpful in maintaining therapeutic levels is to:

  a. increase the dosage.

  b. change the route of administration.

  *c. decrease the dosage.

  d. withhold the medication.

  Reference: p. 404

9. The balance of extracellular fluid is handled by the kidneys through the tubular reabsorption of:

  a. potassium.

  b. calcium.

  c. hydrogen.

  *d. sodium.

  Reference: p. 404

10. The renal tubular epithelium regulates the acid-base balance in the body by:

  *a. the absorption of bicarbonate and excretion of ammonia and hydrogen.

b. reabsorption of water and ammonia in the collecting tubules.

c. the absorption of hydrogen and excretion of ammonia and bicarbonate.

d. the retention of hydrogen ions.

Reference: p. 405

11. The enzyme catalyst that assists with the renal acid-base regulation is:

a. ADH

b. angiotensin II

c. renin

*d. carbonic anhydrase

Reference: p. 405

39
Diuretics

1. The action of a diuretic is essentially the promotion of the excretion of:

   a. potassium

   b. chloride

   *c. sodium

   d. calcium

   Reference: p. 406

2. Carbonic anhydrase inhibitors influence what site to produce its therapeutic action?

   *a. Proximal tubule

   b. Distal tubule

   c. ascending loop of Henle

   d. descending loop of Henle

   Reference: p. 406

3. Because electrolytes are excreted with the fluid when diuretics are taken, a common problem found in patients on diuretics is the depletion of:

   *a. potassium.

   b. chloride.

   c. sodium.

   d. calcium.

   Reference: p. 407

4. If your patient is experiencing hypokalemia, you would expect that he/she is exhibiting the following symptoms:

   a. hyperactive reflexes, and insomnia.

   *b. lethargy and muscle cramps.

   c. bounding, rapid pulse.

   d. heart block and slow pulse.

   Reference: p. 407

5. Dichlorphenamide, a carbonic anhydrase inhibitor, is used frequently in the treatment of:

   a. respiratory failure.

   b. renal failure.

   *c. open-angle glaucoma.

   d. simple edema.

   Reference: p. 407

6. Your patient, 72 year old Mrs. G., has been admitted to your ICU with the diagnosis of acute congestive heart failure. Her drug regime includes Lanoxin .125 mg, and Lasix 40 mg has been ordered. Your nursing actions include:

   *a. fall risk precautions.

   b. weekly weights.

   c. frequent checks of CBCs.

   d. restrictions on the intake of fruit juices.

   Reference: p. 408

7. The only route that Glycerin (Glyrol is given is:

   a. IV.

   *b. PO.

   c. IM.

   d. sq.

   Reference: p. 411

8. The diuretic that is used only for the treatment of acute glaucoma is:

   a. Glycerin (Glycerol.

   *b. Isosorbide (Ismotic.

   c. Mannitol (Osmitrol

   d. Amiloride (Midamor)

   Reference: p. 412

9. In general, appropriate nursing activities for those on diuretics include all except:

   a. Document I&O on every shift.

   b. Check the electrolyte levels frequently.

   c. Caution the patient against eating licorice.

   *d. Warn the patient that a daily weight loss of 5 pounds is not unusual.

   Reference: p. 412

10. An important instruction for your patient taking a loop diuretic is:

   a. "It is important to take your diuretic every day without fail."

   *b. "Report any dizziness and ringing in your ears right away."

   c. "Report any weight loss to your practitioner."

   d. "Take Immodium if you experience any abdominal pain or diarrhea."

   Reference: p. 411

11. The chief use for osmotic diuretics is:

   a. treatment of congestive heart failure.

   b. prophylaxis against pulmonary edema.

   *c. prevention of acute renal failure.

   d. routine treatment of edema.

   Reference: p. 411

12. The fact that the osmotic diuretics have an overall osmotic effect makes it a helpful drug in all of these instances *except*:

   *a. epilepsy.

   b. cranial injuries.

   c. congestive acute glaucoma.

   d. neurosurgery.

   Reference: p. 411

13. Osmitrol (Mannitol is given only by what route?

   a. PO

   b. IM

   *c. IV

   d. SQ

   Reference: p. 412

14. Your patient, Mr. Smith, is taking Spironolactone (Aldactone. While he is taking this medication, you check his electrolytes frequently to detect:

   a. hypokalemia

   *b. hyperkalemia

   c. hypercalcemia

   d. hyponatremia

   Reference: p. 415

15. Mr. Smith has asked you, "are there any over-the-counter medications that I should *not* take while I am taking Aldactone?" You reply:

   a. "There are no problems with any over the counter medications."

   b. "You should not take any products that contain magnesium, such as milk of magnesia."

   *c. "Salicylates will reverse the effects of your Aldactone."

   d. "Certain anti-acids will potentiate the effects of Aldactone."

   Reference: p. 416

16. Mr. Smith asks you if he should take potassium while he is taking Aldactone. Your *best* reply is:

   a. "That idea sounds like a good one-I'll get an order for potassium for you."

   b. "No-don't worry about that unless your physician decides you need supplementation."

   c. "Yes-you will need a source of potassium supplementation.

   *d. " No-the diuretic that you are taking does not pull potassium from your body."

   Reference: p. 416

17. While caring for a patient who is on Amiloride (Midamor, what labs should the nurse monitor?

   a. Glucose, Na, serum creatinine.

   b. SGOT, SGPT, PTT.

   *c. BUN, K, Na.

   d. Hgb, HCT, CBC.

   Reference: p. 415

18. What condition is a *contraindication* to the use of thiazide diuretics?

   *a. Allergy to sulfonamides.

   b. Hepatic cirrhosis

   c. History of kidney stones.

   d. Presence of diabetes insipidus.

   Reference: p. 419

19. Thiazides react with all but:

   a. oral anticoagulants.

   b. oral hypoglycemics.

   c. vasopressors.

   *d. aminoglycosides.

   Reference: p. 419

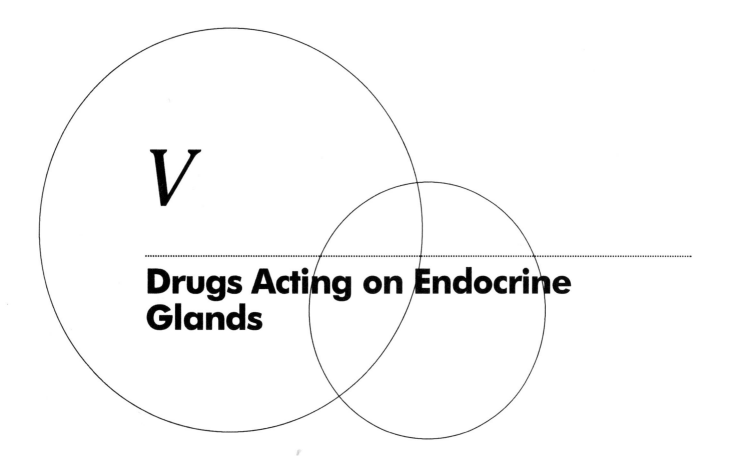

V

Drugs Acting on Endocrine Glands

40
The Endocrine Glands: A Review

1. Inhibition of the production of a given hormone by an endocrine gland by the elevation of it's plasma concentration is termed:
   a. positive feedback.
   b. metabolic transformation.
   *c. negative feedback.
   d. molecular binding.
   Reference: p. 433

2. Factors known to stimulate the release of antidiuretic hormone (ADH), thereby enhancing water reabsorption from the renal tubules include all of the following *except*:
   a. emotional stress.
   b. pain sensations.
   c. increased plasma osmolality
   *d. increased ECF volume.
   Reference: p. 424

3. Expected assessment findings in the patient with inappropriate ADH syndrome, include all of the following *except*:
   a. concentrated urine.
   *b. intense thirst.
   c. low serum osmolality.
   d. hyponatremia.
   Reference: p. 425

4. The hormone of the adenohypophysis (anterior lobe of the pituitary) known to promote the synthesis and release of triiodothyronine (T_3) and thyroxine (T_4) is:
   a. prolactin.
   b. corticotropin.
   c. somatotropin.
   *d. thyrotropin.
   Reference: p. 427

5. The hormones that functions to increase the rate of metabolism, total heat production, and oxygen consumption by the body tissues are:
   a. ADH; vasopressin.
   b. prolactin; luteinizing hormone.
   *c. triiodothyronine (T_3); thyroxine (T_4).
   d. insulin; glucagon.
   Reference: p. 429

6. A hyperplastic disorder of the thyroid gland, most commonly resulting from iodine deficiency is:
   a. myxedema.
   b. cretinism.
   c. thyrotoxicosis.
   *d. goiter.
   Reference: p. 429

7. An expected finding in Hester Locke, a 55 year old female with myxedema (adult hypothyroidism) would be:
   a. restlessness.
   *b. cold intolerance.
   c. tremor.
   d. high pulse pressure.

   Reference: p. 429

8. An expected finding in a patient with an increased parathormone serum levels secondary to a parathyroid adenoma is:
   a. hypocalcemia.
   *b. hypercalcemia.
   c. hyperphosphatemia.
   d. decreased calcitonin.

   Reference: p. 430

9. All of the following factors promote glucagon secretion except:
   a. fasting.
   *b. hyperglycemia.
   c. exercise.
   d. hypoglycemia.
   Reference: p. 431

10. The major effect of insulin on cellular metabolism is to:

   a. inhibit incorporation of amino acids hepatic protein.

   b. stimulate the breakdown of triglycerides.

   c. activate enzymes that stimulate glycogenolysis.

   *d. facilitate glucose transport across cell membranes.

   Reference: p. 431

11. Observable symptoms associated with hypoglycemia, such as sweating, palpitation, anxiety, and weakness, are due to the effects of:

   a. pancreatic somatostatin.

   b. pancreatic polypeptide.

   *c. epinephrine.

   d. insulin.

   Reference: p. 432

12. Henrietta Matisse, 37 years old, is diagnosed as having a pheochromocytoma. The nurse would expect to assess the patient for all of the following clinical and metabolic manifestations of this disorder except:

   a. hyperglycemia.

   *b. bradycardia.

   c. profuse sweating.

   d. elevated blood pressure.

   Reference: p. 433

13. The hormone that plays a major physiological role in maintaining fluid and electrolyte balance by promoting the renal reabsorption of sodium and the secretion of potassium and hydrogen is:

   *a. aldosterone.

   b. cortisol.

   c. antidiuretic hormone.

   d. melano-liberin.

   Reference: p. 434

14. Clinical manifestations of excessive glucocorticoid (cortisol) production associated with Cushing's syndrome include all of the following except:

   a. elevated blood sugar.

   *b. thickening of the skin.

   c. moon face; buffalo hump.

   d. muscular wasting.

   Reference: p. 435

15. Jillian Durbin, 27 years old, is receiving replacement therapy for treatment of her Addison's disease. An assessment finding that would indicate inadequate replacement therapy would be:

   a. hypercalcemia, hypophosphatemia.

   b. decrease serum protein, hypercalcemia.

   d. increased osmolality, hypernatremia.

   *d. hyponatremia, hyperkalemia.

   Reference: p. 435

41
Hypophysial Hormones

1. Because of the effect of ACTH on glucocorticoid production it needs to be used with extreme caution in all of the following situations except:

   a. in patients with ocular herpes simplex.

   b. in patients with systemic fungal infections.

   c. in patients receiving immunizations.

   *d. in patients with allergic bronchitis.

   Reference p. 437

2. The nurse should caution patients on long-term ACTH therapy to follow the physicians guidelines for withdrawal of the drug:

   a. to avoid rebound glucocorticoid production

   b. to prevent psychic changes (e.g, mood swings).

   *c. to minimize effects of adrenal insufficiency.

   d. to control sodium and water retention.

   Reference p. 437

3. Health teaching for patients receiving corticotropin injection (ACTH) should emphasize the need to immediately report:

   a. weight loss.

   *b. infections.

   c. transitory dizziness.

   d. insomnia.

   Reference p. 437

4. A synthetic hormone used to treat hypopituitary dwarfism by stimulating increase in linear bone growth is:

   a. histrelin acetate (Suppelin).

   b. nafarelin (Synarel).

   *c. somatren (Protropin).

   d. demopressin acetate (Concentraid).

   Reference p. 438

5. Which of the following hormones would the nurse expect to be utilized to reverse the excessive water loss associated with diabetes insipidus?

   a. intermediate acting insulin

   *b. vasopressin (Pitressin Synthetic).

   c. oxytocin, parenteral (Pitocin).

   d. corticotropin injection (ACTH).

   Reference p. 440

6. A drug the nurse would expect to be prescribed as an adjunct to therapy to control hemorrhage associated with esophageal varices is:

   *a. vasopressin (Pitressin Synthetic).

   b. oxytocin, parenteral (Pitocin)

   c. desmopressin acetate (DDAVP)

   d. ergonovine (Ergotrate)

   Reference p. 440

7. A patient develops abdominal distention post-surgically for which the attending physician prescribes vasopressin injection (Pitressin Synthetic) 5 U IM. Prior to administering the medication the nurse should:

   a. assess the pulse and blood pressure.

   b. assess the cardiac sounds and rhythm.

   *c. assess bowel sounds and abdominal girth.

   d. assess for tinnitus and double vision.

   Reference p. 441

8. Critical surveillance measures in the patient who is receiving an IV infusion of oxytocin for the induction of labor would include close monitoring for the development of:

   a. jaundice.

   *b. water intoxication.

   c. dehydration.

   d. urinary retention.

   Reference p. 443

9. The primary use of ergonovine (Ergotrate) is for:

   a. the management of incomplete abortion

   b. the management of the second stage of labor.

   *c. severe, recurrent, debilitating migraine headaches.

   d. the management of postpartum hemorrhage.

   Reference p. 444

42
Thyroid Hormones and Antithyroid Drugs

1. The laboratory value that is assessed to determine the adequacy of therapy in patients receiving liothyronine sodium—T$_3$ (Cytomel) is:

a. free thyroxine index.

*b. TSH level.

c. resin uptake of radioactive T$_3$.

d. radioimmunoassay for T$_3$ and T$_4$.

Reference: p. 448

2. In the patient taking thyroid hormones, the nurse should be particularly alert to the possibility of drug toxicity related to:

a. estrogens.

b. oral hypoglycemics.

*c. digitalis glycosides.

d. diuretics.

Reference: p. 449

3. Nursing assessment for Turner Blue, a 39 year old insulin-dependent diabetic who is beginning therapy for hypothyroidism with levothyroxine (Synthroid), would focus on observations for:

a. mild nervousness and sweating.

*b. an increased need for insulin.

c. early signs of hypoglycemia.

d. bradycardia and hypotension.

Reference: p. 449

4. Health teaching for patients taking thyroid hormones for hypothyroidism should emphasize the need:

a. for daily monitoring of temperature.

b. for testing urine for glucose and albumin.

*c. to continue therapy indefinitely.

d. taking the medication at night.

Reference: p. 450

5. The clinical benefits of antithyroid drugs may not be experienced for several weeks following initiation of therapy because of:

a. occurrence of a compensatory increase in TSH.

*b. effects of previously formed thyroid hormones.

c. a time dependent saturation of receptor sites.

d. the half-life delays attaining effective serum levels

Reference: p. 450

6. The laboratory value should the nurse should expect to monitor closely in the patient being treated for hyperthyroidism with propylthiouracil is the:

a. granulocyte count.

b. thrombocyte count.

*c. prothrombin time.

d. capillary fragility test.

Reference: p. 451

7. Because of the possibility of interference with the effects of the antithyroid drug, health teaching for patients taking these agents should emphasize avoiding over-the-counter preparations containing:

a. calcium.

b. potassium.

c. vitamin K.

*d. iodides.

Reference: p. 451

8. Health education of patients receiving radioactive sodium iodide-I (Iodotope) for hyperthyroidism should include discussion of all of the following *except:*

*a. the need for special radiation precautions.

b. the possible need for thyroid replacement.

c. the need to repeat thyroid function studies.

d. the possible insidious onset of hypothyroidism.

Reference: p. 452

9. The physician prescribes saturated solution of potassium iodide (SSKI) 0.6 ml 4 times a day diluted in fruit juice for a patient prior to a thyroidectomy. In discussing the purpose of ther-

apy, the nurse explains to the patient that it is given to:

a. elevate the potassium level quickly.

*b. reduce vascularity of the thyroid gland.

c. bind circulating thyroid hormones.

d. enhance elimination of thyroid hormones.

Reference: p. 452

43
Parathyroid Drugs, Calcitonin, and Calcium

1. To reverse the the bone decalcification of Paget's disease in an elderly male patient, the physician prescribes calcitonin, human (Cibacalcin) 0.5 mg/day SC 3 days a week. To determine the adequacy of the patient's response to drug therapy, the nurse will monitor his serum level of:

   *a. alkaline phosphatase.

   b. magnesium.

   c. inorganic phosphorus.

   d. aspartate transaminase.

   Reference: p. 456

2. The expected effects of etidronate (Didronel) that a physician prescribes for a patient with paraplegia secondary to a spinal cord injury is:

   a. increased urinary excretion of alkaline phosphate.

   *b. reduction in the rate of bone turnover.

   c. blockage of the hypercalcemic action of PTH.

   d. replacement of deficient calcium stores.

   Reference: p. 457

3. In patients taking oral calcium salts for the treatment of calcium deficiency states, intestinal absorption of the drug will be enhanced by taking:

   a. vitamin A

   b. vitamin B.

   c. vitamin C.

   *d. vitamin D.

   Reference: p. 458

4. A particularly useful drug used in patients with hypercalcemia and hypercalciuria secondary to advanced neoplasms who are unresponsive to conventional therapy is:

   a. calcium citrate (Citracal).

   b. etidronate (Didronel).

   *c. plicamycin (Mithracin).

   d. aluminum carbonate gel (Basaljel).

   Reference: p. 458

5. A physician recommends that a post-menopausal patient take OTC supplemental oral calcium salts to decrease the risk of osteoporosis. Of the following that are available, which one contains the greatest percentage of calcium?

   a. calcium gluconate

   *b. calcium carbonate

   c. dicalcium phosphate

   d. calcium lactate

   Reference: p. 459

6. To increase utilization of oral calcium patient instructions should include advising the patient to take it:

   a. with a glass of water at bedtime.

   b. with the a meal, preferably supper.

   *c. a half hour before or 1-1.5 hours after meals.

   d. with a glass of milk or serving of yogurt.

   Reference: p. 459

44
Antidiabetic and Hyperglycemic Agents

1. In the patient receiving an intermediate acting insulin (NPH) insulin at 7:15 am, the nurse is aware that the risk for a hypoglycemic reaction is greatest:

   a. prior to the noon meal.

   *b. before supper.

   c. at bedtime.

   d. around 2 am.

   Reference p. 461

2. The patient with hypoglycemia secondary to insulin therapy is likely to exhibit:

   a. increased urination, fatigue, headache.

   *b. sweating, nervousness, confusion.

   c. excessive food and water intake, .

   d. Kussmaul respirations, "fruity" odor to the breath.

   Reference p. 462

3. The nurse administers a combination of regular insulin 15 U and isophane insulin suspension (NPH) 40 units SC to a patient with Type I diabetes around 7:15 am. How soon after the injection should the patient plan to eat breakfast?

   *a. 30 minutes

   b. 90 minutes

   c. 2 hours

   d. 3 hours

   Reference p. 463

4. Health teaching for the patient with insulin-dependent diabetes taking a combination of regular insulin and intermediate (NPH) insulin should include instructions to:

   a. shake both vials vigorously, draw them up in the syringe.

   *b. draw-up the regular before NPH insulin in the same syringe.

   c. withdraw the insulin from the vials before first injecting air.

   d. avoid using the NPH insulin if it appears cloudy.

   Reference p. 463

5. A patient is admitted with a diagnosis of diabetic ketoacidosis for which the physician prescribes an IV of normal saline with regular insulin added. The nurse's is aware that the effects of the insulin given may be altered because there is:

   a. a time related deterioration of the insulin.

   *b. adsorption of the insulin by the plastic tubing.

   c. hyperkalemia accompanying the ketoacidosis.

   d. a high level of hydrogen ions in the blood

   Reference p. 463

6. Health education of the patients with insulin dependent diabetes includes preparing them to assume responsibility for self-care. Which of the following statements by a patient indicates a need for further education?

   a. "I will systematically rotate insulin injection sites."

   b. "I'll store my insulin vial in a cool place when traveling."

   *c. "I will take additional insulin before my tennis game."

   d. "I'll inject the insulin into the subcutaneous fat."

   Reference p. 463

7. The nurse correctly informs the patient taking glyburide (Micronase) that the it lowers blood sugar by:

   a. stimulating gluconeogenesis by the liver.

   b. redistributing insulin to muscle cells.

   *c. enhancing insulin release from beta cells.

   d. increasing the rate of CHO breakdown.

   Reference p. 463

8. Which one of the following oral antidiabetic agents would be classified as "short acting"?

   a. chlorpropamide

*b. tolbutamide

c. glyburide

d. glipizide

Reference p. 464

9. The nurse would expect to monitor patients who develop a hypoglycemic response secondary to chlorpropamide (Diabenese) closely for at least:

a. 12—24 hours.

b. 1—2 days.

c. 2—4 days.

*d. 3—5 days.

Reference p. 464

10. Patients taking oral antidiabetic agents (sulfonylureas) should be warned that alcohol ingestion may elicit:

a. a hyperglycemic effect.

*b. a disulfiram-like reaction.

c. excessive CNS depression.

d. an anaphylactic reaction.

Reference p. 465

11. Because of displacement from protein binding sites resulting in an enhanced hypoglycemic effect, which of the following should the patient taking chlorpropamide (Diabenese) be taught to avoid?

a. antibiotics

*b. salicylates

c. H$_2$ receptor antagonists

d. glucocorticoids

Reference p. 465

12. A nurse reviews the use of glucagon injection for a hypoglycemic response with an insulin-dependent diabetic patient and his care-taker. The caretaker should be taught that if there is no response following the initial glucagon injection it may repeated in:

*a. 20 minutes.

b. 40 minutes.

c. 60 minutes.

d. 90 minutes.

Reference p. 466

13. Health education for patients with diabetes for whom oral antidiabetic drugs have been prescribed should include instructions to:

a. limit exercise to 1-2 hours a day.

*b. avoid excessive sunlight exposure.

c. avoid acetaminophen intake.

d. avoid changing positions rapidly.

Reference p. 466

45
Adrenal Corticosteroids

1. The principal action of the mineralcorticoids (aldosterone) is upon:
   *a. electrolyte metabolism
   b. carbohydrate metabolism.
   c. the immune system.
   d. the sex hormones.
   Reference: p. 469

2. Under what circumstances might the principal action of aldosterone be desirable?
   *a. The patient with hyponatremia.
   b. The dehydrated patient.
   c. The patient with congestive heart failure.
   d. The edematous patient.
   Reference: p. 469

3. The only available mineralocorticoid available at present is:
   a. Aminoglutethimide (Cytadren).
   b. Triamcinolone (Aristocort).
   *c. Fludrocortisone Acetate (Florinef).
   d. Mometasone (Elocon).
   Reference: p. 469

4. Prior to initiating mineralocorticoid therapy, all of the baseline data listed below is needed except:
   a. weight
   b. blood pressure
   c. electrolyte levels
   *d. CBC
   Reference: p. 477

5. Mineralocorticoid therapy is used primarily in the treatment of:
   a. Cushing's Syndrome.
   b. Parathyroidism.
   c. Systemic Lupus Erythematosus.
   *d. Addison's Disease.
   Reference: p. 469

6. The actions of glucocorticoids include all of the following except:
   a. increased protein catabolism.
   b. decreased inflammation reaction.
   *c. sodium excretion.
   d. interference with the release of histamine.
   Reference: p. 469

7. Glucocorticoids are often used to treat:
   a. respiratory distress syndromes.
   *b. inflammatory disorders.
   c. metastatic carcinomas.
   d. renal failure.
   Reference: p. 469

8. A severe adverse reaction to the glucocorticoids is:
   a. azotemia.
   b. muscle spasm.
   *c. osteoporosis.
   d. anorexia.
   Reference: p. 477

9. When educating your patient about corticosteroids, you include all of these statements except:
   a. "Be sure to eat potassium containing foods every day."
   b. "Your condition may worsen at first, so you will need to work with your doctor and adjust the dosage as needed."
   c. "When your course of therapy is finished, we will decrease your dosage gradually, then discontinue the drug."
   *d. "You will need to increase your intake of sodium."
   Reference: p. 478

10. A what point in a 24 hour period do corticosteroids least suppress adrenal activity?
    *a. 6 AM
    b. 12 PM
    c. 6 PM

d. 12 Midnight

Reference: p. 478

11. When giving corticosteroids to a pediatric patient, an important nursing action specific to this patient is:

    a. to review the patient's diet with the parents.

    b. to monitor for signs of hyperglycemia.

    c. to instruct the parents that therapy is begun with high doses.

    *d. to monitor the child's weight and height.

    Reference: p. 477

12. An important instruction to the parents of a child on long-term corticosteroid therapy is:

    a. "Check your child frequently for joint swelling."

    b. "Any vision problems, such as blurring, are transitory and will go away as therapy continues."

    *c. "Do not let your child receive immunizations while taking corticosteroids."

    d. "Don't be concerned if your child develops a fever, illness is not unusual in childhood."

    Reference: p. 477

13. Contraindications to glucocorticoids include all *except*:

    a. peptic ulcer.

    b. active tuberculosis.

    c. herpes simplex.

    *d. rheumatoid arthritis

    Reference: p. 471

14. Long term steroid therapy may lead to all of the following *except*:

    a. round face.

    b. striae.

    *c. muscle wasting.

    d. weight gain.

    Reference: p. 477

15. Which labs are important during adrenal steroid therapy?

    *a. T4, CBC, electrolytes, liver function.

    b. Urine studies, renal function tests, creatinine levels.

    c. Cholesterol levels, bone scans, KUB.

    d. ABG, platelet studies, PTT.

    Reference: p. 479

46
Estrogens

1. The actions of estrogen include all *except*:
   a. endometrial thickening.
   *b. increased bone resorption rate.
   c. decreased serum cholesterol.
   d. closure of the epiphyses.
   Reference: p. 482

2. Hazards of estrogen use include:
   a. congestive heart failure.
   *b. gall bladder disease
   c. spontaneous bone fractures.
   d. immunosuppression.
   Reference: p. 482

3. Estrogens are given cyclically or with progestin in order to reduce the incidence of:
   a. Mammary carcinoma.
   b. Withdrawal bleeding.
   c. Thromboembolic complications.
   *d. Endometrial carcinoma.
   Reference: p. 482

4. Your instructions to your patient concerning drug interactions should include these drugs:
   *a. Coumadin and insulin.
   b. Versed and INH.
   c. Antispas and Valium.
   d. Aspirin and Flexeril.
   Reference: p. 485

5. As you take your patient's history, what would alert you that estrogen is contraindicated for her?
   a. Complaints of excessive bleeding during menstruation.
   b. The presence of polycystic breast disease.
   *c. A history of thromboembylotic disease.
   d. Severe episodes of diaphoresis at night.
   Reference: p. 485

6. Your menopausal patient is taking estrogen because of a familial history of hip fracture. What concurrent therapy would you expect to also recommend?

   a. Fluoride supplementation.
   b. Vitamin D 500 U daily.
   c. Calcitonin 50 IU daily.
   *d. Calcium 1.5 g daily.
   Reference: p. 481

7. Your patient should contact her physician if she experiences the following symptom:
   a. Vaginal bleeding when cycling the medication.
   b. Weight loss.
   c. Nausea early in therapy.
   *d. Depression.
   Reference: p. 486

8. Progestins are useful in the treatment of all of the conditions listed below *except:*
   a. Endometriosis
   *b. Threatened abortion.
   c. Amenorrhea.
   d. Endometrial carcinoma.
   Reference: p. 481

9. A common vaginal problem that occurs during both estrogen and progestin therapy is:
   a. Increased dryness.
   b. Pruritis.
   *c. Candida.
   d. Monilia.
   Reference: p. 488

10. Your instructions to your patient taking progestin would include:
    a. "You can expect your weight to fluctuate quite a bit until your body adjusts to this medication."
    b. "You need to be sure to eat food high in potassium."
    c. "Report any urticaria around the injection site immediately."
    *d. "Report any changes in your vision to your physician."

    Reference: p. 488

47 Drugs Used in Fertility Control

1. The most frequently employed and most effective means of preventing pregnancy in fertile women are:

   a. spermicidal foams, gels, creams.

   b. progesterone contraceptive IUDs.

   *c. steroid contraceptives.

   d. diaphragm and spermicidal combinations.

   Reference: p. 490

2. As compared to estrogen-progesterone combinations, the progestin-only ("mini-pill") oral contraceptive:

   a. has a higher degree of effectiveness.

   *b. has fewer adverse effects.

   c. is taken only half of the month.

   d. causes paralysis of sperm.

   Reference: p. 490

3. The mechanism of action of combination estrogen-progestin oral contraceptives include all of the following *except:*

   a. interference with follicular maturation.

   b. inhibition of the process of ovulation.

   c. make the endometrium unfavorable to implantation.

   *d. increased fallopian tube peristaltic activity.

   Reference: p. 492

4. The most common gastrointestinal side-effect experienced by women taking oral contraceptive agents is:

   a. diarrhea.

   b. flatulence.

   c. abdominal cramps.

   *d. nausea.

   Reference: p. 492

5. The nurse should instruct the patient taking oral contraceptives for birth control that if she misses a dose to:

   a. abstain from sexual intercourse for at least one week.

   b. take the next scheduled dose and use supplementary contraception.

   *c. take the missed dose as soon as she remembers or take two doses the next day.

   d. double the prescribed dose for 4 days and use another contraceptive method.

   Reference: p. 492

6. Of the following conditions that a patient reports in their health history, the one that would be a contraindication to the use of estrogen-progesterone oral contraceptive agents is:

   a. peptic ulcer disease

   *b. thrombophlebitis

   c. rheumatoid arthritis

   d. allergic dermatitis

   Reference: p. 493

7. Risks of cardiovascular side-effects to estrogen therapy are increased significantly in women over 35 years of age who:

   a. consume alcohol.

   b. maintain a high fat diet.

   *c. smoke cigarettes.

   d. exercise minimally.

   Reference: p. 493

8. Health teaching for patients taking oral contraceptives who desire to get pregnant should include instructions to stop drug and use an alternative means of birth control for:

   a. 1 month.

   b. 2 months.

   *c. 3 months.

   d. 4 months.

   Reference: p. 494

9. The woman who has an IUD progesterone contraceptive device (Progestasert) is at increased risk for developing:

a. endometrial proliferation.

b. endometrial cancer.

*c. pelvic inflammatory disease.

d. long term ovulatory suppression.

Reference: p. 494

10. A patient being prepared for a levonorgestrel implant contraceptive system asks the nurse how long the effects of the implant will last. The nurses response is based on the knowledge that that implants need to be replaced every:

a. 2 years.

*b. 5 years.

c. 7 years.

d. 9 years.

Reference: p. 495

11. As single agents, or in combination with another drug, all of the following are used to stimulate ovulation *except*:

*a. medrosyprogesterone.

b. clomiphene.

c. gonadorelin acetate.

d. urofollitropin.

Reference: p. 495

12. In addition to its use in the induction of ovulation, human chorionic gonadotropin (Pregnyl) is used in the treatment of:

a. precocious puberty.

b. prostatic cancer.

*c. cryptorchidism.

d. migraine headaches.

Reference: p. 499

48
Androgens and Anabolic Steroids

1. The term "anabolic" refers to the particular action of:

   *a. growth of skeletal muscle.

   b. promotion of sodium excretion.

   c. decreased sebaceous gland activity.

   d. decreased vascularization of the skin.

   Reference: p. 502

2. One of testosterone's systemic effects includes:

   a. excretion of potassium.

   *b. cessation of bone growth.

   c. dry skin.

   d. subcutaneous fat deposits.

   Reference: p. 502

3. Uses for anabolic steroids include all *except*:

   a. Replacement therapy for pituitary dysfunction.

   b. Stimulation of bone growth in osteoporosis.

   *c. Stimulation of an increase in muscle mass.

   d. Palliative therapy for inoperable breast cancer.

   Reference: p. 502

4. Contraindications to the use of testosterone include a history of:

   *a. Myocardial infarction.

   b. Gall bladder disease.

   c. Bleeding disorders.

   d. Thyroid disorders.

   Reference: p. 505

5. Hypercalcemia can become a problem for those on anabolic steroids. The symptoms of hypercalcemia include all *except*:

   a. constipation.

   b. loss of muscle tone.

   c. polyuria.

   *d. anorexia.

   Reference: p. 505

6. If a patient develops symptoms suggesting that hypercalcemia has developed during androgen therapy, the nurse needs to counsel the patient to:

   a. remain in bed to avoid injury.

   *b. drink copious fluids to avoid kidney stones.

   c. reduce the dosage of the medication.

   d. discontinue the medication.

   Reference: p. 505

7. Periodic lab tests that are important for the patient taking anabolic steroids include:

   a. Renal function tests and BUN.

   *b. Liver function tests and serum cholesterol.

   c. T4 and PTT.

   d. Glucose tolerance and electrolytes.

   Reference: p. 506

8. Ms. G. has been placed on testosterone therapy for treatment of her breast cancer. In teaching her about anabolic steroids, all of the statements below are true *except*:

   a. "If you have trouble with stomach upsets while you are taking this medication, take the pills with food."

   b. "You will need lab work periodically while you are taking this medication."

   c. "If you notice extra weight gain and swollen ankles at night, you may need a prescription for a diuretic."

   *d. "The changes such as extra hair growth will disappear when you stop taking the drug."

   Reference: p. 506

9. Androgens interact with:

   *a. oral anticoagulants.

   b. antibiotics.

   c. antidepressants.

   d. adrenergic blockers.

   Reference: p. 505

10. Two drugs that decrease the action of androgens are:

   a. Darvon and Motrin.

  *b. Seconal and Dilantin.

   c. Zantac and Periactin.

   d. Tensilon and Cogentin.

  Reference: p. 505

11. Proscar is used for the treatment of:

   a. osteoporosis

  *b. benign prostatic hyperplasia.

   c. metastatic breast cancer.

   d. acquired aplastic anemia.

  Reference: p. 506

12. Danazol (Danocrine) is used primarily for the treatment of:

   a. Hypercalcemia.

  *b. Endometriosis

   c. Hirsutism.

   d. Prostatic cancer.

  Reference: p. 507

13. Contraindications to the use of Danazol include:

   a. Hyperthyroidism.

  *b. Chronic renal failure.

   c. Glaucoma.

   d. Ulcerative colitis.

  Reference: p. 507

NOTES

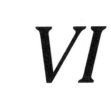

VI

Drugs Acting On Gastrointestinal Function

49
Gastrointestinal Physiology: A Review

1. Which of the following occurs as a result of vagal (parasympathetic) stimulation?
   a. urge to defecate.
   b. contraction of GI sphincters.
   c. decreased secretion of gastric juice.
   *d. increased GI motility/secretion.
   Reference: p. 511

2. *Intrinsic factor*, secreted by the parietal cells of the stomach, is essential to the intestinal absorption of:
   a. vitamin B_6
   b. vitamin C and D.
   c. vitamin K.
   *d. vitamin B_{12}.
   Reference: p. 513

3. The major digestive enzyme secreted by the gastric glands is:
   a. trypsin.
   b. amylase.
   *c. pepsin.
   d. lipase.
   Reference: p. 513

4. Several drugs are absorbed directly from the stomach including:
   a. nitroglycerine, digitalis.
   *b. alcohol, aspirin.
   c. antacids, H_2 receptor antagonists.
   d. vitamin B_{12}, vitamin K.
   Reference: p. 513

5. Absorption of nutrients, vitamins, minerals, water and electrolytes occurs primarily in the:
   a. terminal ileum.
   b. ileum and jejunum.
   *c. duodenum and jejunum.
   d. stomach and duodenum
   Reference: p. 513

6. Lack of bile or pancreatic lipase may impair the absorption of:
   a. vitamins B_6 and B_{12}.
   *b. vitamins A, D, E, K.
   c. ferrous compounds.
   d. vitamin C.
   Reference: p. 516

50
Antacids, Antiulcer Drugs

1. A patient admitted to an acute care facility for treatment of peptic ulcer disease asks the nurse why an antibiotic as part of the therapeutic regimen. The nurse's answer is based on an understanding of research findings that indicate:

   a. antibiotics prevent secondary infection.

   b. antibiotics increase gastric mucous secretion.

   *c. *Helicobacter pylori* causes peptic ulcer disease.

   d. antibiotics block the secretion of pepsin.

   Reference: p. 523

2. A patient is diagnosed as having an active peptic ulcer for which his physician prescribes cimetidine (Tagamet) and magnesium hydroxide. The nurse should advise the patient to notify the physician if he develops:

   a. constipation.

   b. nausea.

   *c. diarrhea.

   d. changed taste.

   Reference: p. 520

3. Prior to being diagnosed with peptic ulcer disease, a patient has been taking sodium bicarbonate to relieve symptoms of epigastric distress. The nurse advises the patient that long-term therapy with this substance should be avoided because of the increased risk of:

   a. abdominal distention.

   *b. systemic alkalosis.

   c. dehydration.

   d. renal stones.

   Reference: p. 520

4. The antacid of choice for a patient with COPD and congestive heart failure being treated for gastric hyperacidity would be:

   a. aluminum hydroxide/magnesium carbonate liquid (Gaviscon)

   b. calcium carbonate/magnesium hydroxide liquid (Di-Gel).

   c. aluminum hydroxide/magnesium hydroxide liquid (Maalox).

   *d. magaldrate liquid (Riopan Plus).

   Reference: pgs. 518—522

5. A physician prescribes an aluminum hydroxide/magnesium hydroxide combination liquid (Maalox Plus) for a patient with a suspected duodenal ulcer. Which of following conditions that the nurse discovers when reviewing the patient's health history is a possible contraindication to its use?

   a. congestive heart failure

   b. high blood pressure

   c. spastic colon

   *d. renal insufficiency

   Reference: p. 523

6. A patient with alcoholic gastritis and reflux esophagitis is admitted to the emergency department with complaints of acute abdominal pain. The physician prescribes aluminum hydroxide/magnesium hydroxide/simethicone liquid (Mylanta II) 30 ml to be given immediately. The nurse correctly informs the patient that the the drug will take effect:

   *a. immediately.

   b. in 15 minutes.

   c. in 45 minutes.

   d. in about one hour.

   Reference: p. 519

7. By raising the gastric pH, antacids bring about their effects through:

   a. inhibition of gastrin release by the antrum.

   *b. inhibition of the proteolytic activity of pepsin

   c. "coating" of the mucosal barrier of the stomach.

   d. increasing lower esophageal sphincter tone.

   Reference: p. 523

8. Health teaching for the patient for whom a aluminum hydroxide/magnesium hydroxide combination liquid (Maalox Plus) has been prescribed for a long-term therapy should include instructions to take the antacid:

   a. every 4 hours around the clock.

   b. between meals and at HS.

   *c. 1 and 3 hours after meals and at HS..

   d. 1 hour before meals and at HS.

   Reference: p. 524

9. An antacid the nurse would expect to be used to treat hyperphosphatemia associated with advanced renal failure is:

   a. calcium carbonate (Tums).

   b. magaldrate (Riopan).

   *c. aluminium phosphate gel (Phosphagel).

   d. magnesium hydroxide (Milk of Magnesia).

   Reference: p. 523

10. For a patient with a duodenal ulcer, a physician prescribes sucralfate (Carafate) 1 g four times a day for 8 weeks. The nurse would instruct the patient to take the medication:

    a. with meals and at HS.

    *b. 1 hour prior to meals and at HS.

    c. with an antacid 4 times a day.

    d. after meals and at HS.

    Reference: p. 524

11. The nurse would inform the patient taking sucralfate (Carafate) that a common side effect experienced is:

    a. insomnia.

    b. nausea.

    c. frequent burping.

    *d. constipation.

    Reference: p. 524

12. Health education for a patient is taking omeprazole (Prilosec) for severe erosive esophagitis includes all of the following instructions *except*:

    a. take the drug on an empty stomach.

    b. take antacids concomitantly.

    *c. discontinue if GI upset occurs.

    d. do not open, chew, crush the capsule.

    Reference: p. 525

13. Which of the following drugs would the nurse expect to be prescribed concomitantly with an NSAID to prevent gastric ulceration?

    a. charcoal (CharcoCaps)

    b. bismuth subsalicylate (Pepto-Bismol)

    *c. omeprazole (Cytotec)

    d. simethicone (Gas-X)

    Reference: p. 526

51
Digestants, Gallstone Solubilizing Agents

1. Health teaching for the patient who is receiving glutamic acid HCL for achlorhydria should include instructions:

    a. to keep the tablets refrigerated.

    *b. to keep the tablets in a dry place.

    c. to keep the tablets in a dark bottle.

    d. to avoid exposing the tablets to heat.

    Reference: p. 529

2. The nurse should instruct the patient who is receiving pancrelipase (Viokase) to take the drug:

    a. after meals with warm liquids.

    *b. during the meal.

    c. before meals with water.

    d. after the evening meal.

    Reference: p. 529

3. Prior to administering pancrelipase (Viokase), nursing interventions should include assessing the patient for history of:

    a. allergic response to iodine containing drugs.

    b. peptic ulcer disease or achlorhydria.

    *c. hypersensitivity to beef or pork products.

    d. indigestion following ingestion of fat.

    Reference: p. 529

4. A laboratory test the nurse will expect to monitor routinely in the patient receiving chenodiol (Chenix), a gallstone-solubilizing agent, is:

    *a. serum aminotransferase (ALT).

    b. serum bilirubin.

    c. alkaline phosphatase.

    d. creatinine phosphokinase.

    Reference: p. 530

5. The nurse would expect that the monoctanoin (Moctanin) prescribed for a patient with cholesterol gallstones in the biliary tract to be administered:

    a. orally, 3 times a day in divided doses.

    b. intramuscularly 2 times a day.

    c. by continuous IV therapy for 24 hours.

    *d. into the common bile duct continuously.

    Reference: p. 531

6. The effects of of ursodiol-ursodeoxycholic acid (Actigall) is mediated through:

    *a. the suppression of hepatic synthesis/secretion of cholesterol, inhibited cholesterol absorption.

    b. the provision of enzymatic activity for the digestion of CHO, protein, and fat.

    c. facilitating the conversion of pepsinogen to pepsin and provision of an optimal pH.

    d. increasing the volume of low-viscosity bile flow.

    Reference: p. 531

52

Laxatives

1. A patient suffering from chronic simple constipation asks the nurse which laxative would be the "safest and most natural." Which of the following of the nurses responses, based on her knowledge of the most "physiologic" type of laxative known to be available, is correct?

   a. "A hyperosmolar laxative, as Glycerin."

   b. "A lubricant type laxative, as Mineral Oil."

   *c. "A bulk-forming laxative, as methylcellulose."

   d. "A fecal softening agent, as Docusate Sodium."

   Reference: p. 533

2. The risk of vitamin A, D, E, and K deficiency is greatest with the use of laxatives classified as:

   a. bulk-forming (methylcellulose).

   *b. lubricant (mineral oil).

   c. saline/osmotic (magnesium citrate).

   d. stimulant (bisacodyl).

   Reference: p. 534

3. The nurse would include all of the following in her health teaching for the patient taking a bulk-forming laxative except:

   *a. "It can be taken indefinitely without consulting your physician."

   b. "Take it mixed in a large glass of water; drink a second one."

   c. "It will take about 3 days before results are experienced."

   d. "Increase whole grains, raw vegetables and prunes in your diet."

   Reference: p. 534

4. A patient with congestive heart failure develops constipation associated with excessively hard, dry stools secondary to prescribed limitations in exercise and water intake. Which of the following laxatives would the nurse expect to be prescribed?

   a. magnesium citrate (Citro-Nesia)

   b. sodium phosphate/biphosphate (Phospho-Soda)

   c. bisacodyl (Dulcolax)

   *d. docusate calcium/diocytl calcium (Dialose)

   Reference: p. 535

5. A condition revealed in the patient's health history that would indicate a contraindication to the use of magnesium citrate is :

   a. hepatitis.

   b. hypothyroidism.

   c. diabetes.

   *d. renal impairment.

   Reference: p. 536

6. Which of the following would the nurse expect to be used in the treatment of portal-systemic encephalopathy (hepatic precoma and coma) to help reduce the patient's blood ammonia levels?

   a. magnesium hydroxide (Milk of Magnesia)

   b. bisacodyl (Dulcolax)

   *c. lactulose (Cephulac)

   d. castor oil (Alphamul)

   Reference: p. 536

7. The nurse correctly instructs a patient being prepared for a barium enema by taking the prescribed polyethylene glycol-electrolyte solution (GoLYTELY):

   a. that there is no need to fast prior to taking the solution.

   b. to discontinue the solution after the first bowel movement.

   c. that it will not cause abdominal cramping or bloating.

   *d. that a bowel movement occurs in 1 hour after the first dose.

   Reference: p. 536

8. As a treatment to promote a return to a normal pattern of bowel evacuation in a patient confined to a bed or wheelchair because of paraplegia, the doctor prescribes a bisacodyl (Dulcolax) rectal suppository 15 minutes after

breakfast. After the insertion of the suppository the nurse expects to place the patient on the toilet in:

*a. 15 minutes.

b. 90 minutes.

c. 2 hours.

d. 4 hours.

Reference: p. 537

53
Antidiarrheal Drugs

1. Locally acting absorbant drugs for the symptomatic relief of mild diarrhea and widely available in OTC preparations are:

   a. paregoric.

   b. loperamide.

   *c. kaolin, pectin.

   d. antiseptic/astringents.

   Reference: p. 539

2. An 8 month old child with acute diarrhea, vomiting, and fever is admitted to a pediatric outpatient clinic. The nurse expects all of the following are likely to be included in the therapy *except*:

   a. an oral antipyretic, as liquid acetaminophen, to control fever.

   b. obtaining a stool culture to attempt to diagnose the cause.

   c. no solid food intake; frequent small amounts of Pedialyte.

   *d. diphenoxylate HCL/atropine sulfate (Lomotil) 4 ml orally.

   Reference: p. 540

3. Medford Gendorf develops severe diarrhea while vacationing in Mexico and begins self-treatment with large doses of defenoxin HCL/atropine sulfate (Motofen) supplied by a fellow traveler in his tour group. If the drug is taken for a prolonged period of time Mr. Gendorf is at increased risk for developing all of the following *except*:

   a. toxic megacolon.

   b. respiratory depression.

   *c. water intoxication.

   d. urinary retention.

   Reference: p. 540

4. Which of the following drugs would the nurse expect to be prescribed for a patient suffering from chronic diarrhea associated with inflammatory bowel disease?

   *a. loperamide (Imodium)

   b. diphenoxylate HCl/atropine sulfate (Lomotil)

   c. opium tincture, camphorated (Paragoric)

   d. bacterial culture (*Lactobacillus acidophilus*)

   Reference: p. 541

5. In addition to its use for the treatment of acute diarrhea, opium tincture, camphorated (Paregoric) is used in the treatment of:

   a. cocaine withdrawal.

   b. dysmenorrhea.

   *c. neonatal withdrawal syndrome.

   d. migraine headaches.

   Reference: p. 541

6. A physician prescribes a the bulk-forming laxative polycarbophil (Fiberall) for a patient with chronic mild diarrhea. The nurse's explanation to the patient for this seeming contradiction is based on the understanding that the rationale for use of this agent is that it:

   a. absorbs bowel toxins that may be a cause of the diarrhea.

   *b. absorbs excess fecal fluid producing formed stools.

   c. acts locally to sooth the irritated intestinal mucosa.

   d. helps to restore the normal bacterial flora of the bowel.

   Reference: pgs. 535, 543

7. An antidiarrheal agent that is sometimes used to treat diarrhea associated with the use of antibiotics is:

   a. bismuth subsalicylate (Pepto-Bismol).

   b. colloidal activated attapulgite (Rheaban).

   c. opium tincture, camphorated (Paragoric).

   *d. *Lactobacillus acidophilus.*

   Reference: p. 543

54
Emetics and Antiemetics

1. The nurse explains to the patient with chronic diabetic gastroparesis (gastric stasis) that the mechanism of action of the prescribed metoclopramide (Reglan) is to:

    a. reduce smooth-muscle contraction by acting on the gut wall.

    b. depress the vomiting mechanism in the brain stem.

    *c. stimulate upper GI motility, decrease normal inhibitory tone.

    d. interfere with the vestibular activation of the CTZ.

    Reference: p. 544

2. The nurse teaching emergency care measures to mothers attending parenting classes instructs them to avoid giving ipecac syrup in all of the following situations *except* when the child has:

    a. become semicomatose from taking sleeping pills.

    *b. just taken 15 tablets of her prenatal iron pills.

    c. drunk motor oil being saved for recycling.

    d. taken a corrosive lye-based household cleaner.

    Reference: p. 546

3. A nurse giving advice to a mother on the use of ipecac to induce vomiting in situations where it is indicated is instructed to contact an emergency room if the drug does not to induce vomiting within:

    a. 20 minutes after the first dose.

    *b. 20 minutes after the second dose.

    c. 5 minutes after 2 doses.

    d. 10 minutes after the first dose.

    Reference: p. 547

4. A patient who suffers from motion sickness obtains meclizine hydrochloride, an antihistamine, to take prior to a plane trip. The nurse explains to the patient that the mechanism of action of this agent is:

    a. to inhibit peristalsis of the upper gastrointestinal tract.

    *b. to decrease sensitivity of the inner ear vestibular apparatus.

    c. to augment cholinergic activation of the vomiting center.

    d. to decrease anxiety and produce a feeling of drowsiness.

    Reference: p. 547

5. The nurse explains to the patient that a common side effect experienced with meclizine hydrochloride is:

    a. nausea.

    *b. drowsiness.

    c. tinnitus.

    d. constipation

    Reference: p. 547

6. A patient with metastatic ovarian cancer receiving intravenous chemotherapy suffers bouts of severe nausea and vomiting following each treatment. Potent antiemetics that act on the CTZ via a dopaminergic blocking action and are used to treat drug-induced nausea and vomiting are:

    *a. phenothiazines, e.g., prochlorperazine.

    b. anticholinergic agents, e.g., scopolamine.

    c. sedatives, e.g., a barbiturate.

    d. antihistamines, e.g., meclizine.

    Reference: p. 547

7. An activity that the patient who is taking an antiemetic should be instructed to avoid:

    a. prolonged exposure to sunlight.

    b. taking a nature walk alone by a lake.

    c. riding in a car for long periods.

    *d. using power tools such as a saw.

    Reference: p. 547

8. The nurse instructs the patient who's physician has prescribed prochlorperazine (Compazine) for nausea

associated with cancer chemotherapy to avoid drinking their usual evening cocktail because:

a. the possibility of addiction to the drug is increased.

b. the alcohol will neutralize the effect of the antiemetic.

*c. CNS depressants shouldn't be taken with antiemetics.

d. alcohol inhibits the absorption of prochlorperazine.

Reference: p. 547

9. The nurse would anticipate administering benzquinamide (Emete-Con) for nausea and vomiting associated with anesthesia or surgery to the patient:

a. immediately after the patient is fully awakened.

b. when the patient complains of feeling nauseated.

*c. 15 minutes prior to the patient's anticipated awakening

d. at hourly intervals after the patient is fully awake.

Reference: p. 548

10. A physician prescribes dronabinol (Marinol) for a patient who is experiencing nausea and vomiting associated with cancer chemotherapy. Which of the following responses by the nurse to the patient's complaints of "impaired ability to think, paranoid thoughts, nightmares, and tingling in the extremities" is appropriate?

a. "You will need to stop taking the medication immediately."

*b. "These symptoms usually do not last for more than 24 hours."

c. "These symptoms disappear with less frequent doses."

d. "Most likely these are caused by the cancer chemotherapy."

Reference: p. 549

NOTES

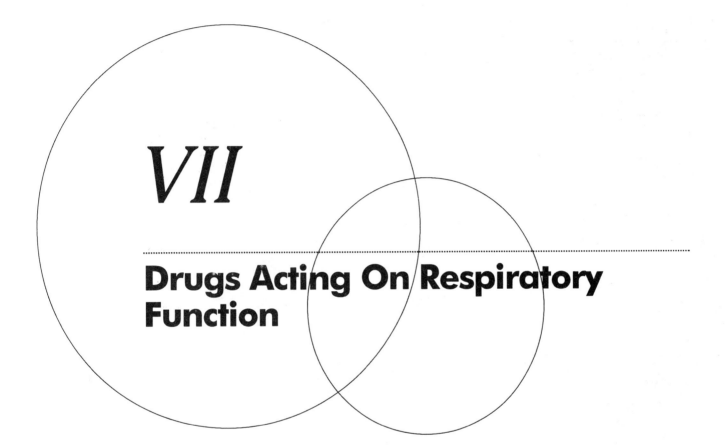

VII

Drugs Acting On Respiratory Function

55 Respiratory Physiology: A Review

1. The cellular utilization of O_2 for oxidative metabolism and the production of CO_2 describes the process of:
   a. transport of gases.
   b. pulmonary exchange of gases.
   c. blood-tissue exchange of gases.
   *d. cellular respiration.
   Reference: 557

2. A major defense against bacterial invasion of the lungs is:
   a. the goblet cells.
   b. ciliated columnar epithelium.
   *c. alveolar macrophages.
   d. hair in the nasal passages.
   Reference: 558

3. Resistence to airflow is greatly affected in bronchial asthma by:
   a. narcosis of the medullary respiratory center.
   b. blood O_2 level, hemoglobin concentration.
   *c. respiratory muscle spasm, mucosal edema.
   d. spasms of the intracostal and diaphragm muscles.
   Reference: 559

4. *Physiological dead space* refers to:
   a. the volume of air in the conducting airways.
   *b. the presence of nonfunctioning alveoli.
   c. potential minute respiratory volume.
   d. potential tidal volume with activity.
   Reference: 559

5. The level of concentration of alveolar PO_2 in the normal individual is equal to:
   a. 50 mm Hg.
   b. 75 mm Hg.
   *c. 100 mm Hg.
   d. 160 mm Hg.
   Reference: 559

6. The rate at which O_2 diffuses from the alveoli into the blood is affected by all of the following *except*:
   *a. the concentration of RBC in the blood.
   b. the ventilation-perfusion ratio.
   c. the partial pressure gradient of oxygen.
   d. the functional surface area of the alveoli.
   Reference: 559

7. All of the following reduce affinity of hemoglobin for O_2 *except*:
   a. increase in erythrocyte 2,3 DPG.
   b. a low serum pH (increased acidity).
   c. increased body temperature.
   *d. a high pH (decreased acidity).
   Reference: 561

8. Carotid and aortic bodies, the peripheral chemoreceptors that function in the control of respiration, are triggered by:
   a. the Hering-Breuer reflex.
   b. increased arterial PO_2.
   *c. low arterial PO_2.
   d. increased arterial pH.
   Reference: 562

56
Antitussives, Expectorants, and Mucolytics

1. The effectiveness of codeine in suppressing cough is mediated through its:

   a. depressant effect on the sensory cortex.

   b. stimulating increased of respiratory fluid output.

   *c. depressant effect on the medullary cough center

   d. local anesthetic effect on stretch receptors.

   Reference: 564

2. Health teaching for the patient for whom an antitussive syrup containing codeine is prescribed should include instructions to:

   a. avoid the concurrent use of antihistamines.

   *b. take the medication in the undiluted form.

   c. drink water after taking the medication.

   d. limit its use to the daytime hours.

   Reference: 564

3. A physician prescribes dextromethorphan (Benylin DM) for a 31 year old patient with a nonproductive, hacking cough that has developed secondary to allergic bronchitis. Nursing instructions relative to taking the drug should emphasize that the 24 hour intake should not exceed:

   a. 60 mg.

   b. 80 mg.

   c. 100 mg.

   *d. 120 mg.

   Reference: 565

4. In which of the following patient conditions would the nurse anticipate the use of an expectorant as part of the therapy?

   *a. obstructive pulmonary disease

   b. lobar pneumonia

   c. severe allergic rhinitis

   d. pleuritis

   Reference: 566

5. Which of the following conditions discovered when eliciting a patients health history would alert the nurse to a contraindication to the use of benzonatate (Tessalon Perles)?

   *a. allergy to local anesthetics

   b. history of hepatic disease

   c. allergy to salicylates

   d. respiratory insufficiency

   Reference: 566

6. The nurse should be alert to the possibility of an adverse drug interaction when guaifenesin is being administered concurrently with:

   a. cardiac glycosides.

   b. anticonvulsants.

   c. NSAIDs.

   *d. anticoagulants.

   Reference: 567

7. Which of the following assessments by the nurse would indicate an effective outcome of expectorant therapy?

   a. increased depth of respiration

   *b. increased sputum clearance

   c. increase in "rattling breath sounds

   d. an increased PCO_2

   Reference: 566

8. A priority nursing intervention in all patient receiving mucolytics, expectorants or antitussives, is:

   *a. monitoring the patient's respiratory status.

   b. providing materials for oral hygiene.

   c. teaching the proper disposal expectorated material.

   d. emphasizing the need for additional fluids.

   Reference: 568

9. The physician prescribes acetylcysteine (Mucomyst) 5ml of a 10% solution by nebulizer four times a day for a patient hospitalized for bronchiectasis complicated by pneumonia. Prior to administering the medication, the patient should be told that they may experience:

a. tinnitus.

b. slight nausea.

*c. an unpleasant odor.

d. throat irritation.

Reference: 569

57
Bronchodilators, Antiasthmatics

Nikos LeChat, 25 years old, is admitted to an acute care medical clinical area for the treatment of an acute asthma attack. After a loading dose of aminophyllin, the physician prescribes a maintenance dose of 0. 8 mg/kg/hr by continues IV infusion.

1. The nurse should observe the patient receiving theophyllin for the side effects of:

   a. slowed pulse and low blood pressure.

   b. constipation and decreased bowel sounds.

   c. difficulty voiding and oliguria.

   *d. palpitations and nervousness.

   Reference: 573

2. Twenty-four hours after IV aminophyllin therapy is initiated, the patient's serum theophyllin level is analyzed. Which of the following represents an optimal drug level?

   a. 7 mcg/ml

   *b. 15 mcg/ml

   c. 25 mcg/ml

   d. 35 mcg/ml

   Reference: 573

3. The nurse should closely observe the patient with a marked elevation of the serum theophyllin level for possible:

   a. severe cardiac slowing.

   b. acute renal failure.

   c. sudden loss of consciousness.

   *d. muscle twitching and seizures

   Reference: 573

4. After the patient's acute asthmatic attack subsides, the physician prescribes an oral anhydrous theophylline preparation (Theo-Dur). The nurse would expect to discontinue the IV theophyllin therapy:

   a. following 4 oral doses of theophyllin

   b. 12 hours after the first oral dose of theophyllin.

   *c. when oral therapy with theophyllin is started.

   d. 24 hours before oral therapy with theophyllin is started.

   Reference: 573

5. The most important factor for the physician to consider in prescribing the correct dosage of of theophyllin (Theo-Dur) for a patient is:

   a. pattern of food intake.

   b. exercise level.

   *c. weight.

   d. age.

   Reference: 573

6. A possible significant adverse effect of oral theophyllin therapy for which the nurse should evaluate the patient is:

   *a. gastric bleeding.

   b paralytic ileus.

   c. renal insufficiency.

   d. allergic dermatitis.

   Reference: 573

7. A patient who is taking theophyllin to control an asthma condition reveals in his personal-social history that he smokes 1 1/2 packs of cigarettes a day. Health instructions should include informing the patient that nicotine alters the drug's effectiveness by:

   a. inhibiting absorption.

   b. decreasing distribution.

   c. inhibiting metabolism.

   *d. increasing elimination.

   Reference: 575

8. Prior to being discharged from the acute care setting, a physician prescribes time release theophyllin (Slo-Phyllin) 250 mg 2 times a day for treatment of a patient's asthma. Health education of the patient should include instructions to:

   a. increase vitamin C or citrus fruit intake.

   b. take the drug 1 hour before meals.

*c limit intake of caffeine in all forms.

d. take supplementary calcium tablets.

Reference: 575

9. Patients with bronchial asthma on long term therapy with oral corticosteroids who's treatment is being changed to inhaled corticosteroids are at increased risk for:

a. renal insufficiency.

b. gastric bleeding.

c. Cushing's syndrome.

*d. adrenal insufficiency.

Reference: 576

10. The nurse should instruct the patient who is taking inhaled corticosteroids and not receiving simultaneous systemic steroids that pulmonary function may not improve for:

*a. 1–4 weeks.

b. 4–6 weeks.

c. 6–8 weeks.

d. 10 weeks.

Reference: 576

11. The physician prescribes beclomethasone (Beclovent) 2 inhalations times a day for a patient with chronic bronchitis. The nurse should instruct the patient that following each inhalation it is important to:

a. lie down for at least 30 minutes.

b. drink 8 ounces of milk or eat a snack.

*c. rinse their mouth with warm water.

d. cough forcefully several times.

Reference: 577

12. Which of the following agents would the nurse expect the physician to prescribe as a preventive agent for the patient with exercise induced bronchospasm (asthma)?

a. flunisolide

b. ipratropium

c. triamcinolone

*d. cromolyn sodium

Reference: 578

NOTES

VIII

Anti-infective and Chemotherapeutic Agents

58
Anti-infective therapy: General Considerations

1. *Bactericidal antibiotics* are capable of:
   *a. Weakening the cell walls of the microbes.
   b. Inhibition of nucleic acid metabolism.
   c. Interference with cell metabolism.
   d. Interference with cell division.
   Reference: 584

2. The action of *bacteriostatic antibiotics includes:*
   *a. Interference with cell metabolism.
   b. Weakening of the cell walls of the microbes.
   c. Rupture of cell walls.
   d. Destruction of organisms.
   Reference: 584

3. Which statement best states the rationale for antibiotic therapy against a particular infection?
   a. Antibiotic therapy is not begun until the causative microorganism is identified by a laboratory.
   b. Sensitivity studies are essential before any antibiotic therapy is begun.
   c. Sensitivity studies are not necessary for effective therapy-culture results are sufficient.
   *d. An initial antibiotic selection can be made using patient history and symptoms as a basis for the decision.
   Reference: pgs. 584, 585

4. Prophylactic use of antibiotics is appropriate in these instances:
   a. The presence of kidney stones.
   b. Burn patients.
   *c. Exposure to meningococcal meningitis.
   d. Chemotherapy with antineoplastic drugs.
   Reference: p. 586

5. Mrs. Smith, who suffers from subacute mitral endocarditis receives prophylactic antibiotic treatment against group A streptococcal infection. What antibiotic is her physician most likely to prescribe?

*a. Penicillin G entids.
   b. Doxycycline (Vibramycin).
   c. Cefazolin (Ancef).
   d. Trimethoprim plus sulfamethoxazole (Septra).
   Reference: p. 586

6. A patient who is taking a prolonged course of prophylactic antibiotics must be monitored for the following symptoms:
   a. Urgency, hematuria
   *b. Diarrhea, perianal or vaginal itching.
   c. Wheezing, maculopapular rash.
   d. Epigastric distress, neurotoxicity.
   Reference: p. 587

7. An organism frequently responsible for superinfections during antibiotic therapy is:
   a. Streptococcus.
   *b. Candida.
   c. E. Coli.
   d. Klebsiella.
   Reference: p. 587

8. A microorganism that is resistant to penicillin is most likely also resistant to:
   *a. cephalosporins
   b. fluroquinolones
   c. antineoplastics
   d. antiprotozoals
   Reference: p. 593

9. Hospital-acquired infections are identified by the name:
   *a. nosocomial infection.
   b. pathologic infection.
   c. penicillinase resistant infection.
   d. colonization
   Reference: p. 593

10. Local and systemic fungal infections are often treated with:

    *a. amphotericin B.

    b. penicillin G.

    c. tetracycline.

    d. vancomycin.

    Reference: pgs. 588–589

11. Antibiotics are divided into broad spectrum and narrow spectrum ranges of antimicrobial activity. Which statement best describes the activity of a wide spectrum antibiotic?

    a. The antibiotic primarily affects one group of microorganisms.

    b. Organisms affected are primarily gram negative organisms plus a number of others, such as neisseria.

    *c. The agent is effective against gram-positive and gram negative organisms.

    d. The most effective antibiotic has a wide spectrum of activity.

    Reference: p. 583

12. The antibiotics that should not be given to patients with impaired renal function include:

    a. penicillins

    b. cephalosporins.

    *c. aminoglycosides

    d. erythromycin

    Reference: p. 593

59
Sulfanomides

1. Conditions usually treated with sulfonamides include all except:

    a. urinary tract infections.

    b. pneumonias.

    *c. tuberculosis infections.

    d. group A hemolytic beta strep infections.

    Reference: p. 595

2. Mr. Young is taking trimethoprim-sulfamethoxazole (Bactrim). What fact in his medical history would alert you to the fact that he may need smaller doses of the medication?

    a. COPD

    b. Addison's disease.

    c. Peptic ulcer

    *d. Impaired renal function.

    Reference: p. 602

3. What labs are important for you to monitor on your patients taking sulfonamides?

    *a. CBC, UA, Liver and Kidney function tests.

    b. Liver and Kidney sonograms, pulmonary function studies, blood gasses.

    c. Liver and kidney function tests only.

    d. LDH, acid Phosphatase, Alkaline phosphatase.

    Reference: p. 599

4. Sulfonamides interact with:

    *a. oral anticoagulants and oral hypoglycemics.

    b. antianemics.

    c. antianginals and antiarrhythmics.

    d. antidepressants.

    Reference: p. 598

5. Your nursing actions for your patient who is taking a sulfonamide and does have reduced kidney function, include:

    *a. Calculation of intake-output ratios every shift.

    b. Administration of 1000cc Ringer's Lactate IV q 12 hours to improve renal flow.

    c. Assessment for signs of intestinal obstruction q shift.

    d. Administration of antacids to increase absorption.

    Reference: p. 603

6. Mrs. Smith, who has a history of repeated urinary tract infections, is taking sulfisoxazole (Gantrisin) for her latest episode of this problem. Your instructions to her would include all except:

    a. "You need to avoid being outside in the sunlight for long periods of time."

    b. "Wipe from front to back after urinating."

    c. "Notify your doctor if you notice unusual bruising."

    *d. "Be careful about drinking extra fluids, as this may decrease the effectiveness of the medication."

    Reference: p. 598

7. Mrs. Smith's urinary tract infections have continued to recur and the physician has decided to change her medication. The sulfonamide he is most likely to pick because of it's usefulness in the treatment of recurring urinary tract infections is:

    *a. Trimethoprim-sulfamethoxazole (Bactrim).

    b. Sulfamethoxazole (Gantanol).

    c. Sulfadiazine (Microsulfon).

    d. Sulfamethizole (Thiosulfil Forte)

    Reference: p. 595

8. Your patient, who has full and partial thickness burns on both legs, is being treated with mafenide (Sulfamylon) for infection. Mafenide is especially effective against:

    a. beta-hemolytic streptococcus.

    b. staphylococcus aureus.

    *c. pseudomonas aeruginosa.

    d. e. coli.

    Reference: p. 599

9. Your patient with a combination of full and partial thickness burns over his forearms is being treated with topically with Mafenide (Sulfamylon). Your nursing actions in the care of this patient include all except:

   a. Administer analgesics before doing dressing changes.

   *b. Cover all burned areas after the Sulfamylon is applied.

   c. Assess for rashes and itching.

   d. Monitor acid-base balance.

   Reference: p. 600

10. The use of Mafenide (Sulfamylon) would be contraindicated in the presence of an allergy to:

    *a. thiazide diuretics.

    b. anticonvulsants.

    c. anticoagulants.

    d. cephalosporin.

    Reference: p. 600

11. The important labs to consider when using Silvadene are:

    a. Blood gases.

    *b. Kidney function tests.

    c. CBC.

    d. PTT.

    Reference: p. 601

12. Besides use in treating urinary tract infections, trimethoprim-sulfamethoxazole (Bactrim) is also useful in the treatment of:

    *a. pneumocystis carinii.

    b. meningococcal meningitis

    c. impetigo

    d. ileus

    Reference: p. 601

13. The sulfonamide that provides relief from dysuria is:

    a. Sulfacetamide (Sulfex)

    b. Sulfamethizole (Thiosulfil Forte).

    *c. Sulfisoxazole and Phenazopyridine (Azo Gantrisin)

    d. Sulfapyridine (Dagenan)

    Reference: p. 601

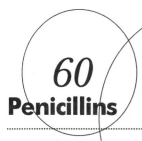

60
Penicillins

1. A frequently used, natural penicillin that is a first-line treatment for infections caused by gram positive bacteria is:

    a. Amoxicillin.

    b. Carbenicillin.

    *c. Penicillin G.

    d. Methicillin.

    Reference: p. 604

2. A major untoward reaction associated with use of the penicillins is:

    a. blood dyscrasias.

    b. ototoxicity.

    *c. hypersensitivity.

    d. renal damage.

    Reference: p. 604

3. The penicillin that is indicated for use against penicillinase-producing Staphylococcus is:

    a. amoxicillin (Amoxil).

    b. carbenicillin (Geocillin).

    c. Penicillin G (Novopen G).

    *d. Methicillin (Staphcillin).

    Reference: p. 611

4. The penicillins act against bacteria by:

    a. Blocking RNA synthesis.

    *b. Interference with the formation of cell walls.

    c. Disruption of internal cellular metabolism.

    d. Repulsion of cellular proteins.

    Reference: p. 604

5. Your patient presents with a severe otitis media with fever and is placed on Amoxicillin 500 mg po q 8 h. Which of the following orders would you question?

    a. "Schedule for an audiogram."

    b. "Encourage fluids to 3000 cc q 24 hours."

    *c. "Tetracycline 500 mg tid po."

    d. "Probenecid 500 mg po qid."

    Reference: p. 612

6. As part of your pretreatment assessment you ask Mrs. Smith, who is to be started on amoxicillin (Amoxil), what other medications she is taking. You are aware that amoxicillin may diminish the effectiveness of:

    a. anticoagulants.

    *b. oral contraceptives.

    c. antacids.

    d. anti-inflammatory agents.

    Reference: p. 612

7. Your instructions to Ms. Smith as she begins her course of oral amoxicillin include all statements except:

    a. "You may take this medication with food if it causes you any GI distress."

    *b. "If you have GI distress, try taking the penicillin with an antiacid."

    c. "Take this medication even after you are feeling well, until all are taken."

    d. "Report any skin rashes to your physician."

    Reference: p. 612

8. You are aware that penicillins can sometimes cause significant adverse reactions. Therefore you carefully monitor your patient on penicillin therapy for all of the following symptoms except:

    a. wheezing.

    b. rash

    *c. tremor.

    d. unusual bruising.

    Reference: p. 612

9. If your patient is allergic to penicillin, s/he may also be allergic to:

    a. tetracyclines.

    *b. cephalosporins.

    c. erythromycin.

    d. sulfonamides.

    Reference: p. 604

10. An order for Imipenem-cilastatin rimaxin) 250 mg IV q 6 has been written for your patient. Your appropriate nursing actions include all of those listed below except:

   a. Administer IV piggyback over 30 minutes.

   b. Monitor kidney function tests.

   c. Assess for thrombophlebitis.

   *d. Monitor for hypertension.

   Reference: p. 614

11. Your patient on prolonged IV sodium or potassium penicillin should have the following periodic labs:

   a. Complete Blood Count.

   b. Prothrombin time.

   *c. Electrolytes.

   d. Creatinine Clearance.

   Reference: p. 605

12. Many organisms become resistant to the effects of penicillins through the manufacture of:

   a. mucopeptides.

   b. increased cell toxins.

   c. mutated RNA.

   *d. beta-lactamase enzymes.

   Reference: p. 604

13. Probenecid is given in addition to Procaine Penicillin G for the treatment of gonorrhea. Probenecid acts by:

   a. Blocking the hepatic breakdown of the penicillin.

   b. Facilitating the excretion of sodium.

   c. Preserving electrolyte balance.

   *d. Prolonging blood levels of penicillins.

   Reference: p. 605

61 Cephalosporins

1. An important difference between first, second, and third generation cephalosporins is that:
   a. The spectrum of antibacterial action is narrower in the third generation than in the first or second generations.
   b. Third generation drugs are less active against gram negative microorganisms.
   *c. The first generation drugs are most effective against gram positive infections.
   d. First generation drugs are the most expensive of the three.
   Reference: p. 617

2. Ms. Brown, who is a 53 year old school teacher, has been placed on cephalexin (Keflex) 500 mg po qid for an infected surgical wound after surgery for a torn knee ligament. You take her health history, keeping in mind that problems may arise if she has a history of:
   a. hepatic failure.
   *b. impaired renal function.
   c. wide angle glaucoma.
   d. hyperkalemia or hyponatremia.
   Reference: p. 625

3. Oral Keflex does not eradicate Ms. Brown's surgical wound infection, which cultures show is caused by Pseudomonas. The physician prescribes another cephalosporin commonly used for bone and joint infections, which is:
   *a. cefonicid (Monocid).
   b. cefamandole (Mandol).
   c. cefmetazol (Zefazone).
   d. cefoxitin (Mefoxin)
   Reference: p. 620

4. What fact in your patient's history would lead you to question an order for cefadroxil (Duricef)?
   *a. an episode of urticaria following injected penicillin.
   b. acute, intermittent porphyria.
   c. cardiac arrhythmias.
   d. intermittent episodes of gout.
   Reference: p. 625

5. Before Ms. Grimm begins taking cefaclor(Ceclor), you teach her about her medication regime, including all of the statements below except:
   a. "You will be taking this medication for at least 10 days; be sure to take it until it is all gone."
   *b. "Take this medication between meals."
   c. "Report any unusual bruising."
   d. "You may become ill again if you abruptly quit taking this drug."
   Reference: pgs. 625—626

6. The cephalosporin often added to dialysis fluid is:
   a. cefaclor (Ceclor).
   b. cefadroxil (Duricef).
   c. cefazolin (Ancef).
   *d. cephalothin (Keflin).
   Reference: p. 618

7. The effects of cephalosporins can be increased and prolonged by concurrent administration of:
   a. Tetracycline.
   b. Phenergan.
   c. Vancomycin.
   *d. Probenecid.
   Reference: p. 625

8. Drug interactions associated with cephalosporins include:
   a. barbiturates.
   b. antihypertensives.
   *c. alcohol.
   d. penicillins.
   Reference: p. 625

9. What alarming adverse reaction would you immediately report to your patient's health care practitioner if the patient is taking one of the cephalosporins?

*a. Diarrhea with blood, pus, or mucus.

b. Painful tongue with white material present.

c. Presence of urinary casts.

d. Recurring headaches.

Reference: p. 626

10. When your patient is taking ceftriaxone (Rocephin), it is important to monitor the following lab work:

a. Liver studies.

*b. Prothrombin times.

c. Urinary glucose.

d. Hemoglobin.

Reference: p. 624

11. Cephalosporins are commonly used in surgical patients for:

a. postoperative wound infections.

*b. surgical prophylaxis in GI surgery.

c. control of wound irritants.

d. empiric therapy based on observed symptoms.

Reference: p. 617

62
Tetracyclines

1. Contraindications to the use of tetracyclines include all of the following *except*:

   a. severe renal impairment.

   *b. glaucoma.

   c. under 8 years old.

   d. pregnancy.

   Reference: p. 631

2. The fact that minocycline (Minocin) is found in high levels in the saliva makes it useful for treatment of:

   a. infection following dental surgery.

   b. gum disease.

   *c. meningitis carriers.

   d. pulmonary diseases.

   Reference: p. 627

3. While taking minocycline (Minocin), you caution your patient taking this drug:

   a. not to take with food.

   b. to avoid diary products.

   c. to avoid exposure to direct sunlight.

   *d. use care in driving or operating machinery.

   Reference: pgs. 629—630

4. Tetracyclines have been found to be useful in the treatment of all *except*:

   a. Intestinal amebiasis.

   *b. Group A Hemolytic Strep infections.

   c. Chlamydial infections

   d. Rickettsial infections.

   Reference: p. 627

5. Your patient is taking Achromycin 250mg po qid and is experiencing some nausea from the capsules. Your advice is:

   a. "Take the drug with a glass of milk."

   b. "Take some Maalox at the same time that you take the pill."

   c. "Take the Achromycin with meals."

   *d. "Instead of 3 large meals, eat 6 small meals and take the Achromycin in between."

   Reference: p. 631

6. Doxycycline (Vibramycin) 300mg IV daily has been ordered for your patient. Appropriate nursing actions include:

   a. checking the history and labs for renal impairment.

   *b. mixing the Vibramycin with 250 ml NaCl and infusing over a 2 hour time period.

   c. cautioning the patient to avoid exposure to direct sunlight.

   d. cautioning the patient not to take the medication with food.

   Reference: p. 628

7. An important instruction for your patient taking demeclocycline (Declomycin) is:

   a. "This drug can be taken with milk."

   b. "Your medication may turn your skin yellow."

   c. "You may notice that you bruise easily while you are taking this drug."

   *d. "You will need to avoid direct sunlight while you are taking Declomycin."

   Reference: p. 628

8. Nalidixic Acid (Neg Gram) is indicated for use in the treatment of:

   a. pseudomonas infections.

   b. most pneumonias.

   *c. urinary tract infections.

   d. meningococcal infections.

   Reference: p. 635

9. Nalidixic Acid (Neg Gram) interacts with:

   a. aminoglycocides.

   b. adrenergics.

   *c. antacids.

   d. digitalis preparations.

   Reference: p. 633

10. Your patient has been placed on norfloxacin (Noroxin) 400 mg bid for her urinary tract infection. Prior to initiating therapy, it is important to check her history for the following:

    a. allergy to penicillin.

    *b. renal failure.

    c. cardiac problems.

    d. peptic ulcer.

    Reference: p. 633

11. Norfloxacin (Noroxin) interacts with all of the following except:

    *a. diuretics.

    b. digoxin

    c. oral anticoagulants.

    d. cyclosporine.

    Reference: p. 633)

12. Ciprofloxacin (Cipro) is useful in treating most bacterial infections *except:*

    a. e. coli urinary infections.

    b. strep infection of the skin.

    c. staphylococcus bone infections.

    *d. chlamydia.

    Reference: p. 634

13. Your pre-therapy assessment of your client who is to be started on ciprofloxacin (Cipro) reveals a history of respiratory problems, including asthma, bronchitis, and COPD. You then review his medication list, keeping in mind that Cipro interacts with:

    *a. theophylline.

    b. inhaled corticosteriods.

    c. anticholinergics.

    d. antihistamines.

    Reference: p. 633

14. Your patient taking quinolones will need to be monitored to detect signs of:

    a. hypotension.

    *b. diplopia.

    c. lethargy.

    d. hematuria.

    Reference: p. 635

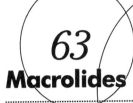

63
Macrolides

1. A major concern with the use of erythromycin is:

   a. frequent, severe adverse drug reactions.

   b. poor absorption and resulting poor bioavability.

   *c. the emergence of resistant microbial strains.

   d. the expense involved in treatment with erythro-mycins.

   Reference: p. 637

2. The most frequently reported adverse reaction with the erythromycins is:

   a. peptic ulcer.

   b. photosensitivity.

   c. renal failure.

   *d. diarrhea.

   Reference: p. 637

3. A common use for erythromycins is the treatment of:

   *a. respiratory infections due to H. influenzae.

   b. meningococcal meningitis

   c. pseudomonas infections.

   d. infections of the G.I. tract due to e. coli.

   Reference: pgs. 637–639

4. Mr. Brown has been placed on E-mycin 333 mg qid po after contracting Legionnaire's disease. Your instructions to him include the statement:

   a. "If you have a problem with GI upset, you may crush the tablet for better absorption."

   b. "You may take this tablet at mealtimes."

   c. "This medicine may be taken with milk."

   *d. "Take this medication on an empty stom-ach."

   Reference: p. 639

5. Before you start Mr. Brown on E-mycin, you review his history and medication list, knowing that E-mycin interacts with:

   *a. oral anticoagulants.

   b. diuretics.

   c. antihistamines.

   d. calcium channel blockers.

   Reference: p. 638

6. When your patient is taking Erythromycin Esto-late (Ilosone), it is important to assess freqently for the following symptoms:

   a. flank pain, anurea.

   *b. right upper quadrant pain, vomiting.

   c. chest pain, diaphoresis.

   d. hypotension, tachycardia.

   Reference: p. 639

7. The best form of erythromycin to give when immediate high blood levels of medication is needed is:

   a. erythromycin ostolate (Ilosone).

   b. erythromycin stearate (Eramycin).

   c. erythromycin ethylsuccinate (E-mycin E.)

   *d. erythromycin gluceptate (Ilotycin Gluceptate).

   Reference: p. 639

8. The use of troleandomycin (Tao) is contraindi-cated in the presence of:

   *a. Liver disease.

   b. Renal impairment.

   c. Cardiac disease.

   d. Pulmonary disease.

   Reference: p. 643

9. Labs that are important during therapy with azithromycin (Zithromax) are:

   a. electrolytes, blood chemistry.

   *b. urinalysis, liver and kidney function.

   c. prothrombin times, thyroid studies.

   d. kidney and liver scans.

   Reference: p.643

10. You have instructed your patient who is taking clarithromycin (Biaxin) to report signs of hema-

tologic toxicity to the prescribing practitioner. These signs include:

a. nausea, diarrhea, headache.

b. dizziness, hearing loss.

*c. sore throat, mucosal ulceration.

d. sensitivity to sunlight, drowsiness.

Reference: p. 643

64
Aminoglycosides

1. The aminoglycoside that is effectively used against tuberculosis is:

   a. penicillin.

   *b. streptomycin.

   c. tetracycline.

   d. tobramycin.

   Reference: p. 648

2. A major limitation in the use of aminoglycosides is that:

   a. parenteral administration of these drugs is impractical.

   b. these drugs are very irritating to the gastric mucosa.

   *c. the possibility of a serious adverse reaction is high.

   d. the cost of these drugs is prohibitive.

   Reference: p. 645

3. Lab reports show that your patient, who is taking amikacin (Amikin), has an increased number of casts in his urine. Your appropriate nursing actions include all except:

   a. contact the practitioner to decrease the dosage.

   b. increase the dosing intervals.

   c. increase the fluid intake.

   *d. give furosemide to increase excretion of the drug.

   Reference: p. 650

4. Peak serum concentrations are used to determine:

   a. the amount of medication absorbed by the body.

   b. hepatic activity in drug metabolism.

   *c. the extent of drug activity.

   d. drug accumulation and toxicity.

   Reference: p. 645

5. Trough serum concentrations are used to determine:

   a. the amount of medication absorbed by the body.

   b. hepatic activity in drug metabolism.

   c. the level of drug activity.

   *d. drug accumulation and toxicity.

   Reference: p. 645

6. Amikacin (Amikin) 500 mg t.i.d. IM has been prescribed for your patient, Mr. C. In performing your history and assessments, you know that it is especially important to assess:

   a. visual acuity

   *b. eighth cranial nerve function.

   c. tenth cranial nerve function.

   d. cardiac function.

   Reference: p. 650

7. Before starting amikacin (Amikin) for Mr. C., you take his health history. You are especially alert for a history of:

   a. hepatic impairment.

   b. cardiac disease.

   *c. renal impairment.

   d. circulatory impairment.

   Reference: p. 650

8. An important lab to obtain before starting an antimicrobial medication on a patient with an infection is:

   a. sodium levels.

   *b. culture and sensitivities.

   c. calcium levels.

   d. prothrombin times.

   Reference: p. 650

9. In taking Mr. C's drug history, you note that he is taking furosemide (Lasix). You notify the physician to suggest a change in the medication combination because:

   a. the aminoglycoside blood levels would tend to be lowered due to the diuretic action of the furosemide.

   b. the aminoglycoside would potentiate the action of the furosemide, possibly causing dehydration.

c. the two interact, causing both to precipitate from the system.

*d. both are ototoxic and the risk of damaged hearing is greater when both are given.

Reference: p. 649

10. During therapy with Amikacin, Mr. C's peak and trough levels of the medication need to be measured at intervals. If you give him his IM Amikacin (Amikin) at 8 a.m. you would draw his peak level at:

*a. 8:30.

b. 9:00.

c. 9:30.

d. 10:00.

Reference: p. 645

11. You schedule Mr C's amikacin (Amikin) IM doses at 8AM and 8PM. You order his trough level to be drawn at:

a. 10:00 AM.

b. 12:45 PM.

c. 7:30 PM.

*d. 7:45 PM.

Reference: p. 645

12. Mr. C. has been on amikacin (Amikin) for ten days, but cultures show that he still needs to remain on the medication. Before continuing the drug, the following tests need to be performed:

a. platelet counts.

b. electrolytes.

c. EEG.

*d. audiogram.

Reference: p. 630

13. Important labs to be monitored throughout therapy with aminoglycosides are:

a. electrolytes, chemistry panels.

*b. liver and kidney function tests.

c. arterial blood gasses.

d. blood clotting tests.

Reference: p. 650

14. Neomycin (Mycifradin) interacts with:

a. benazepril (Lotensin).

b. dextromethorpan (Benylin DM).

*c. digitalis (Digoxin).

d. pilocarpine (ilocar).

Reference: p. 648

15. A course of tobramycin (Tobrex) has been prescribed for your patient to treat her conjunctivitis. Your teaching includes the statement:

a. "Do not take the medication with food."

*b. "Notify your health care practitioner if you develop a sore throat."

c. "Wear a sun screen and protective clothing if you go into direct sunlight."

d. "Do not take any over the counter medications when taking tobramycin."

Reference: p. 648

16. The use of streptomycin is contraindicated in the presence of:

*a. labyrinthine disease.

b. immunizations.

c. gout.

d. rheumatic disorders.

Reference: p. 648

17. Aminoglycosides are best absorbed when given:

a. orally

b. topically

c. by inhalation

*d. parenterally

Reference: p. 645

65
Polypeptides

1. Systemic use of bacitracin (Baciguent) is virtually obsolete because:

    a. the incidence of bacterial resistance is very high.

    b. Baciguent has a brief half-life.

    *c. parenteral administration is highly nephrotoxic.

    d. the cost outweighs the benefits of the drug.

    Reference: p. 653

2. Polymyxins act upon bacteria by:

    a. interference with cell metabolism.

    *b. rupture of the cellular wall.

    c. disruption of RNA functions.

    d. disruption of DNA synthesis.

    Reference: p. 653

3. If given parenterally, the Polymyxins do not reach these tissues:

    a. urinary system.

    b. cardiovascular system.

    c. pulmonary system.

    *d. central nervous system.

    Reference: p. 653

4. The infections that the Polymyxins are most effective against are:

    a. multiply resistant respiratory tract infections.

    *b. severe urinary tract infections.

    c. gastric infections.

    d. joint infections.

    Reference: p. 652

5. Polymyxins are used most widely for the treatment of infections of:

    a. bone tissue.

    b. lymph tissue.

    *c. eye and ear.

    d. nail beds.

    Reference: p. 652

6. Principal adverse reactions to Polymyxins involve these systems:

    a. respiratory and gastric.

    b. cardiac and musculoskeletal.

    c. lymphatic and vascular.

    *d. renal and neural.

    Reference: p. 653

7. Contraindications to the use of colistimethate (Coly-Mycin M) include all except:

    *a. concurrent use of anticoagulants.

    b. severe renal failure.

    c. concurrent use of aminoglycosides.

    d. concurrent use of vancomycin.

    Reference: p. 654

8. Colistin sulfate (Coly-Mycin S) is used in the treatment of:

    *a. diarrhea and external otitis.

    b. scabies and conjunctivitis.

    c. tuberculosis and influenza.

    d. burns and renal disease.

    Reference: p. 654

9. The polypeptide used most frequently for topical application is:

    a. colistimethate (Coly-Mycin M).

    *b. bacitracin (Baciguent).

    c. colistin Sulfate (Coly-mycin S).

    d. polymyxin B Sulfate (Aerosporin).

    Reference: p. 652

10. The most helpful nursing action to take to protect a client against renal toxicity is to:

    a. monitor serum creatinine levels.

    b. give the medication on around the clock schedule.

    *c. maintain good hydration.

    d. avoid parenteral administration.

    Reference: p. 653

11. Your patient, Mr. D., is taking Colistimethate (Coly-Mycin M) 250 mg qid IV. Which order would you question?

    a. "I&O q shift."

    b. "Daily BUN."

    c. "Serum Creatinine before initiating therapy."

    *d. "Procainamide 500mg q 6 h po.

    Reference: p. 653

12. When giving polymyxin to a patient with meningitis, which route must you use?

    a. Deep intramuscular injection.

    b. Inhalation.

    *c. Intrathecal.

    d. Intravenous.

    Reference: p. 655

13. Your nursing actions for the patient receiving Aerosporin parenterally include:

    a. close observation the level of consciousness.

    *b. frequent assessment of your patient's grip strength.

    c. monitoring of the auditory status.

    d. assessment of the patient's cardiac status.

    Reference: p. 656

14. Baseline data needed to detect adverse effects that may occur with an antiinfective otic agent include all except:

    a. vital signs.

    b. tympanic membrane integrity.

    c. hematologic function.

    *d. electrolyte status.

    Reference: pgs. 656–659

64
Aminoglycosides

1. The aminoglycoside that is effectively used against tuberculosis is:
   a. penicillin.
   *b. streptomycin.
   c. tetracycline.
   d. tobramycin.
   Reference: p. 648

2. A major limitation in the use of aminoglycosides is that:
   a. parenteral administration of these drugs is impractical.
   b. these drugs are very irritating to the gastric mucosa.
   *c. the possibility of a serious adverse reaction is high.
   d. the cost of these drugs is prohibitive.
   Reference: p. 645

3. Lab reports show that your patient, who is taking amikacin (Amikin), has an increased number of casts in his urine. Your appropriate nursing actions include all except:
   a. contact the practitioner to decrease the dosage.
   b. increase the dosing intervals.
   c. increase the fluid intake.
   *d. give furosemide to increase excretion of the drug.
   Reference: p. 650

4. Peak serum concentrations are used to determine:
   a. the amount of medication absorbed by the body.
   b. hepatic activity in drug metabolism.
   *c. the extent of drug activity.
   d. drug accumulation and toxicity.
   Reference: p. 645

5. Trough serum concentrations are used to determine:
   a. the amount of medication absorbed by the body.
   b. hepatic activity in drug metabolism.
   c. the level of drug activity.

*d. drug accumulation and toxicity.
   Reference: p. 645

6. Amikacin (Amikin) 500 mg t.i.d. IM has been prescribed for your patient, Mr. C. In performing your history and assessments, you know that it is especially important to assess:
   a. visual acuity
   *b. eighth cranial nerve function.
   c. tenth cranial nerve function.
   d. cardiac function.
   Reference: p. 650

7. Before starting amikacin (Amikin) for Mr. C., you take his health history. You are especially alert for a history of:
   a. hepatic impairment.
   b. cardiac disease.
   *c. renal impairment.
   d. circulatory impairment.
   Reference: p. 650

8. An important lab to obtain before starting an antimicrobial medication on a patient with an infection is:
   a. sodium levels.
   *b. culture and sensitivities.
   c. calcium levels.
   d. prothrombin times.
   Reference: p. 650

9. In taking Mr. C's drug history, you note that he is taking furosemide (Lasix). You notify the physician to suggest a change in the medication combination because:
   a. the aminoglycoside blood levels would tend to be lowered due to the diuretic action of the furosemide.
   b. the aminoglycoside would potentiate the action of the furosemide, possibly causing dehydration.

c. the two interact, causing both to precipitate from the system.

*d. both are ototoxic and the risk of damaged hearing is greater when both are given.

Reference: p. 649

10. During therapy with Amikacin, Mr. C's peak and trough levels of the medication need to be measured at intervals. If you give him his IM Amikacin (Amikin) at 8Am, you would draw his peak level at:

*a. 8:30.

b. 9:00.

c. 9:30.

d. 10:00.

Reference: p. 645

11. You schedule Mr C's amikacin (Amikin) IM doses at 8AM and 8PM. You order his trough level to be drawn at:

a. 10:00 AM.

b. 12:45 PM.

c. 7:30 PM.

*d. 7:45 PM.

Reference: p. 645

12. Mr. C. has been on amikacin (Amikin) for ten days, but cultures show that he still needs to remain on the medication. Before continuing the drug, the following tests need to be performed:

a. platelet counts.

b. electrolytes.

c. EEG.

*d. audiogram.

Reference: p. 630

13. Important labs to be monitored throughout therapy with aminoglycosides are:

a. electrolytes, chemistry panels.

*b. liver and kidney function tests.

c. arterial blood gasses.

d. blood clotting tests.

Reference: p. 650

14. Neomycin (Mycifradin) interacts with:

a. benazepril (Lotensin).

b. dextromethorpan (Benylin DM).

*c. digitalis (Digoxin).

d. pilocarpine (ilocar).

Reference: p. 648

15. A course of tobramycin (Tobrex) has been prescribed for your patient to treat her conjunctivitis. Your teaching includes the statement:

a. "Do not take the medication with food."

*b. "Notify your health care practitioner if you develop a sore throat."

c. "Wear a sun screen and protective clothing if you go into direct sunlight."

d. "Do not take any over the counter medications when taking tobramycin."

Reference: p. 648

16. The use of streptomycin is contraindicated in the presence of:

*a. labyrinthine disease.

b. immunizations.

c. gout.

d. rheumatic disorders.

Reference: p. 648

17. Aminoglycosides are best absorbed when given:

a. orally

b. topically

c. by inhalation

*d. parenterally

Reference: p. 645

65
Polypeptides

1. Systemic use of bacitracin (Baciguent) is virtually obsolete because:
   a. the incidence of bacterial resistance is very high.
   b. Baciguent has a brief half-life.
   *c. parenteral administration is highly nephrotoxic.
   d. the cost outweighs the benefits of the drug.
   Reference: p. 653

2. Polymyxins act upon bacteria by:
   a. interference with cell metabolism.
   *b. rupture of the cellular wall.
   c. disruption of RNA functions.
   d. disruption of DNA synthesis.
   Reference: p. 653

3. If given parenterally, the Polymyxins do not reach these tissues:
   a. urinary system.
   b. cardiovascular system.
   c. pulmonary system.
   *d. central nervous system.
   Reference: p. 653

4. The infections that the Polymyxins are most effective against are:
   a. multiply resistant respiratory tract infections.
   *b. severe urinary tract infections.
   c. gastric infections.
   d. joint infections.
   Reference: p. 652

5. Polymyxins are used most widely for the treatment of infections of:
   a. bone tissue.
   b. lymph tissue.
   *c. eye and ear.
   d. nail beds.
   Reference: p. 652

6. Principal adverse reactions to Polymyxins involve these systems:
   a. respiratory and gastric.
   b. cardiac and musculoskeletal.
   c. lymphatic and vascular.
   *d. renal and neural.
   Reference: p. 653

7. Contraindications to the use of colistimethate (Coly-Mycin M) include all except:
   *a. concurrent use of anticoagulants.
   b. severe renal failure.
   c. concurrent use of aminoglycosides.
   d. concurrent use of vancomycin.
   Reference: p. 654

8. Colistin sulfate (Coly-Mycin S) is used in the treatment of:
   *a. diarrhea and external otitis.
   b. scabies and conjunctivitis.
   c. tuberculosis and influenza.
   d. burns and renal disease.
   Reference: p. 654

9. The polypeptide used most frequently for topical application is:
   a. colistimethate (Coly-Mycin M).
   *b. bacitracin (Baciguent).
   c. colistin Sulfate (Coly-mycin S).
   d. polymyxin B Sulfate (Aerosporin).
   Reference: p. 652

10. The most helpful nursing action to take to protect a client against renal toxicity is to:
    a. monitor serum creatinine levels.
    b. give the medication on around the clock schedule.
    *c. maintain good hydration.
    d. avoid parenteral administration.
    Reference: p. 653

11. Your patient, Mr. D., is taking Colistimethate (Coly-Mycin M) 250 mg qid IV. Which order would you question?

   a. "I&O q shift."

   b. "Daily BUN."

   c. "Serum Creatinine before initiating therapy."

 *d. "Procainamide 500mg q 6 h po.

Reference: p. 653

12. When giving polymyxin to a patient with meningitis, which route must you use?

   a. Deep intramuscular injection.

   b. Inhalation.

 *c. Intrathecal.

   d. Intravenous.

Reference: p. 655

13. Your nursing actions for the patient receiving Aerosporin parenterally include:

   a. close observation the level of consciousness.

 *b. frequent assessment of your patient's grip strength.

   c. monitoring of the auditory status.

   d. assessment of the patient's cardiac status.

Reference: p. 656

14. Baseline data needed to detect adverse effects that may occur with an antiinfective otic agent include all except:

   a. vital signs.

   b. tympanic membrane integrity.

   c. hematologic function.

 *d. electrolyte status.

Reference: p. 656

66
Urinary Antiinfectives

1. Urinary antiinfectives are useful in the treatment of those who:

   a. suffer from severe renal failure and dehydration.

   b. suffer from a variety of infections.

   c. have a history of hepatic disease.

   *d. have an infection that is unresponsive to a first line drug.

   Reference: p. 658

2. 70 year old Mrs. Smith is being started on methenamine (Hiprex) 1000mg qid po for recurrent urinary tract infections. Before you begin to give her this medication, you check her history for:

   *a. hepatic impairment.

   b. Myasthenia Gravis.

   c. labyrinthitis.

   d. cardiac failure.

   Reference: p. 659

3. Your instructions to Mrs. Smith as she begins her treatment with methenamine include:

   a. "Limit your fluid intake, as the medication must become concentrated in the urine."

   b. "It is better to have a catheter in place while your bladder is infected."

   c. "Be sure to notify your doctor if your ears begin to ring."

   *d. "You need to add ascorbic acid to your diet."

   Reference: p. 660

4. You inform Mrs. Smith that the chief action of methenamine (Hiprex) in the bladder consists of:

   a. acidification of the urine.

   *b. generation of formaldehyde.

   c. alkalinization of the urine.

   d. bactericidal action against pseudomonas.

   Reference: p. 660

5. You caution Mrs. Smith that while she is taking methenamine (Hiprex), she will need to avoid:

   a. taking the drug with food.

   b. intake of extra fluid.

   c. taking any over the counter medications.

   *d. a high intake of citrus fruits.

   Reference: p. 660

6. Methenamine hippurate (Hiprex) is especially useful in the treatment of:

   *a. chronic urinary tract infections.

   b. kidney stones.

   c. acute urinary tract infections.

   d. dysuria due to urinary tract infection.

   Reference: p. 659

7. Methenamine (Hiprex) interacts with:

   a. methazolamide (Neptazane).

   b. cefotaxime sodium (Claforan).

   *c. trimethoprim/sulfamethoxazole (Septra).

   d. conjugated estrogen remarin).

   Reference: p. 659

8. The urinary antiinfective that is used also as an antidote for cyanide poisoning is:

   a. cinoxacin (Cinobac).

   b. methenamine mandelate (Mandelamine).

   c. nitrofurantoin (Furadantin).

   *d. methylene blue (Urolene Blue).

   Reference: p. 660

9. A frequent adverse reaction to Nitrofurantoin (Furadantin) is:

   *a. nausea and vomiting.

   b. mental confusion

   c. blurred vision.

   d. constipation.

   Reference: p. 667

10. While your patient is taking nitrofurantoin (Furadantin), you will need to monitor for:

    a. polyuria.

146

b. hypotension.

*c. dyspnea.

d. nystagmus.

Reference: p. 662

11. Nitrofurantoin may cause urinary tract superinfection, especially of the organism:

a. e. coli.

b. candida albicans.

c. staphylococcus aureus.

*d. pseudomonas aeruginosa.

Reference: p. 662

12. An appropriate nursing action for the patient taking nitrofurantoin (Furadantin) is to:

a. caution the patient that the drug may cause discoloration of the urine.

*b. give the medication with meals.

c. instruct your patient that dark glasses should be worn when he/she is outside.

d. warn your patient not to consume alcohol.

Reference: p. 662

13. The urinary antiseptic that also exerts analgesic actions within the urinary tract is:

*a. phenazopyridine yridium).

b. trimethoprim roloprim).

c. cinoxacin (Cinobac).

d. methenamine (Mandelamine).

Reference: p. 664

14. The use of phenazopyridine yridium) is contraindicated in the presence of:

a. hypertension.

b. acute glaucoma.

*c. glomerulonephritis.

d. penicillin allergy.

Reference: p. 664

15. Patients taking nitrofurantoin (Furadantin) should be warned that:

a. irreversible damage to the eighth cranial nerve may occur.

*b. the urine may be discolored.

c. food will delay absorption.

d. pulmonary symptoms may result from long term therapy.

Reference: p. 664

16. Your teaching to the patient taking phenazopyridine yridium includes this statement:

a. "You will need to take this medication on an empty stomach."

*b. "Notify your practitioner if you develop a sore throat or begin to bruise easily."

c. "Avoid drinking milk while you are taking this medicine."

d. "Be sure to use a sunscreen when you go outside."

Reference: p. 664

17. Acetohydroxamic acid (Lithostat) is useful for:

a. treatment of acute urinary tract infections.

b. treatment of chronic urinary tract infections.

c. relief of pain and urinary urgency.

*d. adjunctive treatment of urinary infections.

Reference: p. 665

18. A particular characteristic of urinary antiinfectives is:

*a. the lack of systemic antibacterial activity.

b. high serum concentrations of these medications.

c. rapid excretion by the hepatic route.

d. the lack of toxic effects.

Reference: p. 658

19. A major problem encountered in the treatment of urinary infections is:

a. irreversable kidney damage.

b. development of chronic renal failure.

*c. recurring infections.

d. high cost of treatment.

Reference: p. 658

67
Miscellaneous Antibiotics

1. Atovaquone (Mepron) exhibits activity against:
   a. Mycobacterium tuberculosis
   b. Candida albicans.
   *c. Pneumocystis carinii.
   d. Pseudomonas aeruginosa.
   Reference: p. 667

2. Your instructions to your patient taking atovaquone (Mepron) include the statement:
   a. "Stay out of the sun or wear a sunscreen when you take this medication. "
   b. "Report any unusual bruising to your practitioner. "
   c. "Do not take this medication with milk. "
   *d. "Take this medication with meals. "
   Reference: p. 667

3. Chloramphenicol (Chloromycetin) is the treatment of choice for:
   a. carrier state of typhoid fever.
   b. staphylococcus skin infections.
   c. strep throat infections.
   *d. acute typhoid fever.

   Reference: p. 668

4. A common use for chloramphenicol (Chloromycetin) is:
   *a. local treatment of superficial ocular infections.
   b. typhoid carrier states.
   c. hepatitis B.
   d. tuberculosis.
   Reference: p. 668

5. A serious adverse drug reaction noted with the use of chloramphenicol (Chloromycetin) is:
   a. hepatic failure.
   b. glomerular damage.
   *c. bone marrow depression.
   d. pulmonary damage.
   Reference: p. 668

6. Contraindications for chloramphenicol (Chloromycetin) include:
   a. concurrent administration of an ototoxic drug.
   *b. flu syndrome.
   c. treatment with MAO inhibitors.
   d. hepatic disease.

   Reference: p. 669

7. In assessing your patient for side effects of chloramphenicol (Chloromycetin), which of the following lab studies should you be following?
   a. SGOT, SGPT, Lactic acid dehydrogenase.
   b. HDL, LDL, triglycerides.
   c. electrolyte and chemistry studies.
   *d. blood counts, leukocyte and reticulocyte counts.

   Reference: p. 669

8. Your teaching for your patient on chloramphenicol (Chloromycetin) therapy includes the statement:
   *a. "Be sure to report any unusual bruising to your physician. "
   b. "This drug is especially suited for long-term therapy. "
   c. "You must take this medication on an empty stomach. "
   d. "You do not have to be concerned with side effects after the drug is discontinued. "

   Reference: p. 669

9. When you learn that your patient who will begin chloramphenicol (Chloromycetin) therapy is also diabetic, your next question is:
   a. has your diabetes caused any kidney damage?
   *b. are you taking insulin or an oral hypoglycemic medication?
   c. how well controlled is your diabetes?
   d. do you have any vision problems?
   Reference: p. 670

10. Chloramphenicol (Chloromycetin) interacts with:

    a. prednisone.

    b. persantine.

    c. theophylline.

    *d. erythromycin.

    Reference: p. 671

11. A major concern in the use of lincosamides such as Clindamycin and Lincomycin is:

    a. the development of Clostridium superinfections.

    b. renal damage from crystal formation in the nephrons.

    c. ototoxic reactions, resulting in labyrinthitis.

    *d. diarrhea and pseudomembranous colitis.

    Reference: p. 699

12. Lincosamides are indicated for treatment of infections due to:

    a. pneumocystis carinii.

    b. salmonella typhi.

    *c. penicillin resistant strep.

    d. E. coli.

    Reference: p. 671

13. A medication that has proven to be effective in the treatment of leprosy is:

    a. lincomycin (Lincocin).

    b. clindamycin (Cleocin).

    c. nitrofurazone (Furacin).

    *d. dapsone (Avlosulfon).

    Reference: p. 764

14. Furazolidone (Furoxone) is used for the treatment of:

    a. otic infections.

    b. viral meningitis.

    c. staph epidermis infections.

    *d. protozoal diarrhea.

    Reference: p. 676

15. Furazolidone (Furoxone) interacts with:

    *a. alcohol.

    b. penicillin.

    c. ibuprofen.

    d. diuretics.

    Reference: p. 676

16. Your education for a patient taking furazolidone (Furoxone) includes:

    a. "If you see any change in the color of your urine, be sure to inform your physician. "

    *b. "Avoid eating cheese while you are taking this medication. "

    c. "Report any bruising you experience while you are taking this drug. "

    d. "Avoid standing up or sudden movements, as this drug may cause you to be dizzy. "

    Reference: p. 677

17. Uses for nitrofurazone (Furacin) include:

    a. local application in otitis media.

    b. treatment of streptococcal skin infections.

    c. treatment of stage 3 & 4 decubiti.

    *d. prevention of infection in severe burns.

    Reference: p. 677

18. Novobiocin (Albamycin) is rarely used because of:

    a. extreme nephrotoxic reactions.

    b. high incidence of hepatic damage.

    *c. high incidence of hypersensitivity reactions.

    d. numerous instances of blood dyscrasia.

    Reference: p. 678

19. A prudent nursing action to take while caring for patients during IV infusion of pentamidine entam 300) is:

    a. frequent assessment of respiratory status.

    *b. frequent checks of vital signs.

    c. skin assessments for the presence of urticaria.

    d. frequent checks of urinary output.

    Reference: p. 679

20. Vancomycin is the only drug that is effective in the treatment of:

    *a. penicillin resistant staphylococcal infections.

    b. acute, recurrent urinary tract infections.

    c. the acute symptoms of malaria.

    d. meningococcal meningitis.

    Reference: p. 681

68
Antitubercular Agents

1. Because of GI distress, nausea, anorexia, and diarrhea accompanying its intake, there is an increased risk of poor patient compliance with the administration of:

   a. capreomycin.

   b. streptomycin.

   c. cycloserine.

   *d. para-aminosalicylate.

   Reference: p. 685

2. An antitubercular agent used as an alternative treatment of active tuberculosis in combination with other tuberculostatic drugs when first-line therapy has failed is:

   a. streptomycin.

   b. para-aminosalicylate.

   *c. cycloserine.

   d. ethambutol.

   Reference: pgs. 685-688

Hosteen Nez, a 65 year old native-born American, presents at the Chinle Regional Hospital Outpatient Clinic with complaints of a productive cough, fever, and night sweats. He is admitted to the hospital and, after undergoing a series of tests, is diagnosed as having active pulmonary tuberculosis. He is started on rifampin (Rifadin) 400 mg orally daily and isoniazid (INH) 300 mg /day.

3. Following several weeks of therapy with INH and rifampin, the physician adds ethambutol to a patient's drug regimen for tuberculosis. The nurse's instruction should emphasize the importance of:

   *a. monthly visual function testing.

   b. bimonthly audiometric testing.

   c. liver enzyme testing weekly.

   d. frequent drug serum levels.

   Reference: p. 688

4. In the patient who is taking INH and rifampin concurrently, the nurse would expect to routinely monitor the:

   a. serum potassium level.

   *b. serum liver enzymes level.

   c. serum amylase level.

   d. serum osmolality.

   Reference: p. 691

5. Because of a possible side-effect that occurs with isoniazid therapy, which of the following supplementary nutritional agents would the nurse expect to administer?

   a. vitamin B_{12}

   b. vitamin D

   *c. vitamin B_6

   d. folate

   Reference: p. 692

6. The patient is curious about the action of rifampin on the mycobacterium causing his tuberculosis. The nurses explanation is based on the understanding that rifampin:

   *a. inhibits DNA dependent RNA polymerase.

   b. represses mycobacterium folic acid synthesis.

   c. prevents cell wall synthesis in bacteria.

   d. interferes with the synthesis of RNA.

   Reference: p. 693

7. Health teaching for a patient with tuberculosis who is taking rifampin should include instructing the individual to do all of the following except:

   a. take the drug on an empty stomach with water.

   b. take the drug only once a day in a single dose.

   *c. discontinue the drug when symptoms subside.

   d. report changes in hearing and balance.

   Reference: p. 694

8. Health teaching for the patient taking rifampin should include the nurse informing them that the drug may:

   a. result in increased sputum.

   b. cause photosensitivity.

   c. produce rash in sun exposed skin.

   *d. cause a red-orange urine and sputum.

   Reference: p. 695

9. Health teaching for the patient should include advising them that concurrent use of isoniazid (INH) and alcohol increases the risk of:

a. severe CNS depression.

*b. INH induced hepatitis.

c. developing resistance.

d. rapid drug metabolism.

Reference: p. 697

69
Antimalarial Agents

Lara Sullivan, M.D., a volunteer health care worker for the Friends Society, is planning to spend 2 years in a country in Central America where malaria is known to be endemic. In preparation for the trip, she consults with a physician specializing in infectious diseases who prescribes a combination of hydroxychloroquine Plaquenil) and primaquine phosphate rimaquine) prophylactically.

1. The OTC medication that a patient taking hydroxychloroquine laquenil) should be told to avoid is:

   a. buffered aspirin with caffeine.

   b. multi-vitamin and minerals.

   c. bulk-forming laxatives.

   *d. kaolin and magnesium trisilicate.

   Reference: p. 697

2. Which of the following conditions disclosed in the patient's health history would alert the nurse to a possible contraindication to the use of hydroxychloroquine (Plaquenil)?

   a. osteoarthritis

   *b. G6PD deficiency

   c. severe dysmenorrhea

   d. recurrent bladder infections

   Reference: p. 697

3. The nursing diagnosis that is most likely to apply to the patient taking hydroxychloroquine is:

   a. High risk for altered tissue perfusion eripheral).

   b. High risk for altered comfort related to malaise/temperature fluctuations.

   *c. High risk for sensory/perceptual alterations (visual).

   d. High risk for peripheral neurovascular dysfunction.

   Reference: p. 697

4. For suppression of malaria, the patient will need to understand that the prescribed hydroxychloroquine/primaquine combination should be taken:

   a. for 3 weeks prior to leaving for the high risk area until leaving the area.

   b. from the time of arrival in the high risk area until departure from the area.

   c. for 1 week prior to leaving for the high risk area until 2 weeks after returning.

   *d. for 2 weeks before leaving for the high risk area and for 8 weeks after returning.

   Reference: p. 698

5. Nursing instructions for the patient taking combination hydroxychloroquine/primaquine therapy should emphasize the need for routine monitoring of:

   a. serum electrolytes.

   * b. CBC and hemoglobin.

   c. BUN and creatinine levels.

   d. urine amylase.

   Reference: pgs. 698—701

6. The nurse should explain to the patient that a harmless side effect of hydroxychloroquine therapy is:

   a. an altered sensation of smell.

   b. a lingering metallic taste.

   * c. a yellowish-brown urine color.

   d. a tanned appearance to the skin.

   Reference: p. 699

7. The nurse providing health education for the patient taking combination hydroxychloroquine/primaquine therapy should include instructions to take the drugs:

   a. one hour before meals.

   b. with meals or a large snack.

   * c. one to 2 hours after meals with water.

   d. at bedtime with a glass of water.

   Reference: pgs. 698—701

8. The physician prescribes sulfadoxine and pyrimethamine (Fansidar) for a traveler to an area

where chloroquine resistant falciparum is endemic. A condition in which this combination antimalarial therapy contraindicated is:

a. iron-deficiency anemia.

b. secondary polycythemia.

*c. folate deficiency anemia.

d. rheumatoid arthritis

Reference: p. 703

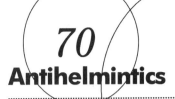

70
Antihelmintics

1. Which of the following nursing diagnoses would apply to the patient with worm infestation?

   a. High risk for sleep pattern disturbance (insomnia).

   *b. High risk for infection transmission.

   c. High risk for fluid volume deficit.

   d. High risk for altered nutrition:More than body requirements.

   Reference: p. 707

2. Health teaching by the nurse relative to preventative measures of helminthic reinfection should include all of the following *except*:

   a. frequent careful handwashing, especially before eating.

   b. daily changes of underwear, towels, bedding.

   *c. intermittent prophylactic courses of anthelminthics.

   d. ingestion of pure water and food.

   Reference: p. 707

3. A 10 year child is diagnosed as having a roundworm (*Ascaris lumbricoides*) infestation for which the physician prescribes mebendazole (Vermox). Health education of the patient should include instructions to:

   a. fast for 24 hours after taking the drug.

   b. repeat the course of therapy in 3 weeks.

   c. consume a fat free diet for 2 weeks.

   * d. chew, crush, or swallow tablets whole.

   Reference: p. 710

4. Fin Picis, a 25 year old male, is being treated for fish tapeworm (*Diphyllobothrium latum)* with niclosamide (Niclocide). Health teaching should include informing the patient that the criterion for cure is a negative stool for worm segments or ova for:

   a. 2 weeks.

   b. 4 weeks.

   c. 6 weeks.

   * d. 12 weeks.

   Reference: p. 711

5. The nurse should instruct the patient to take the prescribed niclosamide (Niclocide):

   a. an hour after meals on an empty stomach.

   *b. with meals and a glass of water.

   c. crushed and dissolved in water .

   d. with an antacid and milk.

   Reference: p. 711

6. The nursing diagnoses that would apply relative to a common side effect that occurs with niclosamide (Niclocide) therapy is:

   *a. High risk for diarrhea.

   b. High risk for hyperthermia.

   c. High risk for disrupted oral mucous membrane.

   d. High risk for altered nutrition (anorexia).

   Reference: p. 711

7. Jasper Sparr, age 5, is seen by his pediatrician for abdominal pain and apathy. He is diagnosed as having pinworm infestation and the physician prescribes piperazine (Antepar). The nurse explains to the patient's mother that the mechanism of action of the drug on the pinworm is:

   *a. causes paralysis of the worm by blocking acetylcholine.

   b. blocks uptake/utilization of glucose by the worm.

   c. inhibits mitochondrial oxidative phosphorylation in the worm.

   d. produces loss of the cell membrane in the worm.

   Reference: p. 712

8. A physician prescribes piperazine (Antepar) for a patient with a pinworm infestation. The drug dosage will be based on the patient's:

   a. quantity of dietary intake.

   b. ideal weight.

   *c. present weight.

   d. age.

   Refererence: p. 712

9. Health teaching for patients taking piperazine (Antepar) for pinworm infestation should emphasize taking the drug as:

   a. a single dose for 2 consecutive days.

   b. two doses on 2 consecutive days; repeat in 1 week.

   *c. a single daily dose for seven consecutive days.

   d. a single dose; repeat in two weeks.

   Reference: p. 712

10. Use of piperazine (Antepar) for the treatment of roundworm or pinworm would be contraindicated in the child with:

   a. iron-deficiency anemia.

   *b. a convulsive disorder.

   c. reactive airway disease.

   d. rheumatic heart disease.

   Reference: p. 712

11. Health teaching by the nurse relative to taking piperazine should include informing the patient or caretaker that a significantadverse reaction to this drug is:

   a. tachypnea.

   b. severe constipation.

   *c. nausea and vomiting.

   d. hallucinations.

   Reference: p. 712

12. A wheat farmer is diagnosed as having rat lungworm (*Angiostrongylus*) for which his physician prescribes thiabendazole(Mintezol). The nurse should caution the patient to:

   a. report an increase in urine output promptly.

   b. discard all expectorated sputum carefully.

   *c. avoid hazardous tasks during therapy.

   d. maintain bedrest during therapy.

   Reference: p. 715

13. Ima Woodsy develops diarrhea, fever, cramps abdominal distention, and greasy stools 14 days following an 4 day hiking trip into a mountainous area. Examination of her stool reveal the cysts of *Giardia lamblia* (giardiasis). The drug most likely to be prescribed for her condition is:

   *a. quinacrine (Atabrine).

   b. quinine sulfate (Quinamm).

   c. pyrimethamine (Daraprim).

   d. hydroxychloroquine laquenil).

   Reference: p. 714

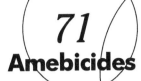

71
Amebicides

1. After his return from the Amazon, a 55 year old anthropologist is diagnosed as having a liver abscess secondary to amebiasis *(Entamoeba histolytica)* infection for which his physician prescribes emetine. The adult dosage of emetine for amebichepatitis is 65 mg given by:

   *a. a single daily injection (SC or IM) for 10 days.

   b. a two times a day injection for 10 days.

   c. oral tablets 4 times a day.

   d. intravenous injection once daily.

   Reference: p. 719

2. The nursing diagnosis that would apply to the patient receiving emetine is:

   a. High risk for hyperthermia.

   *b. High risk for altered comfort (muscle stiffness/pain).

   c. High risk for dysreflexia.

   d. High risk for fluid volume deficit.

   Reference: p. 719

3. A 22 year old female college student presents at the Student Health Center with symptoms of vulvovaginitis. The causative organism is identified as *Trichomonas vaginalis* and the nurse practitioner prescribes metronidazole (Flagyl) 500 mg twice daily for 7 days. Health teaching includes informing the patient of all of the following *except*:

   a. it must be taken by both sexual partners.

   *b. it is best to take it on an empty stomach.

   c. it may leave a metallic taste in the mouth.

   d. alcohol ingestion may elicit a disulfiram-like reaction.

   Reference: pgs. 721—722

4. An 8 year old child hospitalized for the treatment of an anaerobic infection is being treated with IV metronidazole (Flagyl) every 6 hours. The nurse inadvertently repeats the IV metronidazole 2 hours after the previous dose was given. In addition to notifying thechild's physician of the medication error, the nurse would observethe patientcloselyfor:

   *a. incoordination, ataxia, confusion.

   b. hypothermia, shivering, flushing.

   c. tachycardia, low blood pressure.

   d. sweating, nervousness, irritability.

   Reference: p. 721

5. Following 2 weeks of service to victims of a hurricane disaster, a 62 year old male Red Cross supply officer develops dysentery with bloody diarrhea, vomiting, fever, and dehydration. His condition is diagnosed as severe intestinal amebiasis for which his physician prescribes metronidazole (Flagyl). During the time he is taking the drug, the patient should be cautioned to avoid:

   a. aspirin products.

   b. magnesium antacids.

   *c. alcohol.

   d. citrus fruits/vitamin C.

   Reference: p. 721

6. The average daily adult dose of metronidazole (Flagyl) for intestinal amebiasis is:

   a. 500 mg daily orally for 10 day.

   b. 250—500 mg 3 times a day orally for 5 days.

   *c. 500—750 mg 3 times a day for 5 to 10 days.

   d. 1000 mg. once daily orally for 10 days.

   Reference: p. 721

7. A disorder that a patient reports in his medical history that would be an contraindication for the use of metronidazole (Flagyl) is:

   a. hearing loss.

   *b. chronic lymphocytic leukemia.

   c. supraventricular arrhythmia.

   d. rheumatoid arthritis.

   Reference: p. 722

8. Following several days of therapy with metronidazole (Flagyl), the patient complains of very dark urine. Health teaching should include informing the patient:

    a. to increase water intake to 3,000 ml/day.

    b. drink extra fruit juice to acidify the urine

    c. bring a specimen to the clinic for analysis.

  *d. the dark urine is a harmless reaction to the drug.

Reference: p. 722

72
Antifungal Agents

1. A physician prescribes miconazole (Monistat) vaginal cream for a patient with *Candida albicans* vulvovaginitis. The nurse should give all of the following instructions to the patient *except*:

   a. insert the cream high in vagina at bedtime.

   b. avoid sexual intercourse during therapy.

   c. use a sanitary napkin to prevent staining.

   *d. douche before inserting the cream.

   Reference: p. 726

2. Which of the following laboratory tests would the nurse expect to be ordered on a patient with candida vulvovaginitis that isunresponsive to therapy?

   a. culture and sensitivity

   *b. blood sugar

   c. blood culture

   d. electrolyte panel

   Reference: p. 726

3. Frederico Esperaza, a 25 year old Hispanic male, is diagnosed as having systemic coccidioidomycosis and is receiving IV amphotericin B (Fungizone) therapy every other day at the Xanadeaux Outpatient Clinic. The correct procedure for IV administering of amphotericin B is:

   a. as a continuous IV over 2 hour period.

   b. as a continuous IV over 12 hour period.

   *c. as a continuous IV over a 6 hour period.

   d. as an "IV push" over 15 minutes in 2 doses.

   Reference: p. 728

4. A patient receiving IV amphotericin B for disseminated coccidioidomycosis asks, "What the usual length of time of therapyfor my condition? "The nurse correctly responds:

   a. "The usual length of time is 4 weeks. "

   *b. "It usually lasts for several months. "

   c. "Minimally, it will last 9 months. "

   d. "It usually lasts for 12 months. "

   Reference : p. 728

5. The nurse tells the patient being treated with IV amphotericin B that a common side effect experienced with the drug is:

   *a. nausea, vomiting.

   b. skin rashes, itching.

   c. frequent urination, back pain.

   d. constipation, flatulence.

   Reference: p. 728

6. In the patient receiving long term IV amphotericin B therapy, the nurse should plan to closely monitor all of the following *except*:

   a. BUN and creatinine.

   *b. ECG and EEG.

   c. liver function studies.

   d. hearing acuity.

   Reference: p. 729

7. Nursing interventions for the patient receiving IV amphotericin B should include monitoring the person closely for signs and symptoms of:

   a. hyponatremia.

   b. hyercalcemia.

   *c. hypokalemia.

   d. hypomagnesemia.

   Reference: p. 729

8. Health teaching for the patient with a persistent fungal infection of the toenails for which their physician has prescribed griseofulvin (Fulvicin P/G) should emphasize the need for weekly:

   *a. hematologic studies.

   b. liver enzymes.

   c. BUN and serum creatinine.

   d. fasting blood sugars.

   Reference: p. 732

A 4 month old female infant is brought to the pediatrician's office for evaluation. She refuses to take her bottle, is running a slight fever, and her mother has noticed white patches and ulcers on her oral mucous membrane. The physician diagnoses her condition as thrush (oral candida infection).

9. The antifungal drug most often prescribed for acute oral candida infection is:

a. miconazole (Monistat).

b. natamycin (Natacyn).

c. butoconazole (Femstat).

*d. nystatin (Mycostatin).

Reference: p. 736

10. The nurse should instruct the mother that the procedure for the administration of the oral antifungal liquid prescribed for her infant's thrush is to:

a. mix it in 1 ounce of milk, give.

b. place it on the tongue, follow by water.

*c. place half of a dose on each side of the mouth.

d. mix it in 1/2 ounce of water, give.

Reference: p. 736

73
Antiviral Agents

1. A nurse teaching parents attending a program on maintaining their children's health correctly informs them that viral diseases are best managed by administering:

   a. antibacterial antibiotics.

   b. antiviral drugs.

   *c. vaccines and serums.

   d. combination antiviral/antibiotic drugs.

   Reference: p. 738

2. The nurse practitioner caring for a patient with genital herpes lesions prescribes acyclovir (Zovirax) ointment to be applied to the lesions. Health teaching should include informing the patient that:

   a. the drug will eliminate the infection within 10 days.

   b. the drug is not effective against recurrent lesions.

   *c. the drug will not prevent the spread of infection to others.

   d. lesions need to be cultured 5 days after treatment begins.

   Reference: p. 739

3. Health teaching for the patient using topical acyclovir (Zovirax) should include informing them that a common side effect of the drug is:

   a. depigmention.

   *b. burning, stinging.

   c. blistering.

   d. local anesthesia.

   Reference: p. 739

4. A 29 year old patient presents at the Woman's Health Clinic with complaints of painful shallow ulcers on her external genitalia. The nurse practitioner diagnoses herpes genitalis and prescribes acyclovir (Zovirax) 200 mg orally. Health teaching by the nurse should include informing the patient:

   a. to stop treatment when symptoms subside.

   b. treatment will eliminate contagiousness.

   c. treatment will confer immunity to the virus.

   *d. to seek treatment for recurrence promptly.

   Reference: p. 740

5. During an influenza A virus epidemic, a receptionist in an outpatient clinic is repeatedly exposed to patients with type A flu. A day ago she received the influenza Asian (A) vaccine and in addition the clinic physician prescribed amantadine (Symmetrel) 100 mg twotimes a day. The clinic nurse explains that the rationale for this is:

   *a. prophylaxis until her body to builds up antibodies.

   b. to augment the effects of the vaccine.

   c. to prevent infection by another virus.

   d. to prevent a bacterial infection.

   Reference: p. 740

6. The nurse explains to the patient receiving amantadine (Symmetrel) that the mechanism of action of the drug on the virus results from:

   a. neutralizing the effects of viral toxins.

   b. killing the organisms that are present.

   *c. blocking viral replication at an early stage.

   d. inhibiting effects of viral DNA polymerases.

   Reference: p. 740

7. A hospitalized infant is being treated with ribavirin (Virazole) for a lower respiratory tract infection caused by respiratory syncytial virus. In addition to giving the drug as prescribed by a special aerosol generator, nursing interventions would include all of the following except:

   a. assessing fluid status frequently.

   b. closely monitoring the respiratory status.

   c. checking blood pressure often.

   *d. checking deep tendon reflexes frequently.

   Reference: p. 744

8. Following an episode of Pneumocystis carinii pneumonia, a physician prescribes zidovudine (Retrovir) as palliative treatment for a patient with acquired immune deficiency related complex(ARC). The usual dosage is:

*a. 200 mg every 4 hours around the clock.

b. 200 mg 4 times a day at equally spaced intervals.

c. 600 mg 2 times a day at equally spaced intervals

d. 1200 mg once daily at bedtime.

Reference: p. 746

9. The nurse should inform the patient on chronic zidovudine (Retrovir) therapy that common side effects include:

a. drowsiness, prolonged sleeReference

*b. headache, nausea.

c. polyuria, dysuria.

d. vivid dreaming, hallucinations.

Reference: p. 746

10. Nursing care of the patient on on chronic zidovudine (Retrovir) therapy includes monitoring of:

a. liver enzyme studies weekly.

b. BUN and creatinine serum levels.

*c. CBCs with differentials every at 2 weeks.

d. electroencephalographic studies monthly.

Reference: p. 747

11. In reviewing the the drug history of a patient taking zidovudine (Retrovir) the nurse discovers he occasionally takes the following drugs. The one that may impair zidovudine metabolism, thus increasing its potential for toxicity is:

*a. buffered aspirin.

b. aluminum based antacid.

c. vitamin B complex.

d. alcohol based cough syrups.

Reference: p. 747

74
Antineoplastic Agents

1. An oncologist prescribes cyclophosphamide (Cytoxan) 75 mg/m^2 2 times a week for maintenance therapy for Cicily Marins who has carcinoma of the breast. In the patient receiving cyclophosphamide(Cytoxan), the nurse will expect to closely monitor the:

   a. serum estrogen and progesterone levels.

   *b. white blood cell count.

   c. serum uric acid levels.

   d. serum magnesium levels.

   Reference: p. 756

2. Close monitoring for signs and symptoms of syndrome of inappropriate antidiuretic hormone secretion (SIAHS) is a high level priority in patients being treated with cyclophosphamide (Cytoxan) and would include assessment for:

   *a. confusion, agitation.

   b. hallucinations, irritability.

   c. high serum osmolality.

   d. hypernatremia.

   Reference: p. 757

3. The nurse caring for the patient receiving cyclophosphamide (Cytoxan) should be assessing them routinely for the presence of:

   a. hypercalcemia.

   b. hyperglycemia.

   *c. hematuria.

   d. edema.

   Reference: p. 760

4. A nursing intervention that should be implemented in caring for patients receiving cyclophosphamide (Cytoxan) therapy is:

   a. administering the drug with meals or with a large snack.

   *b. maintaining a fluid intake at 3,000 liters/day.

   c. administering the drug at bedtime with an antacid.

   d. limiting intake of high sodium content foods.

   Reference: p. 760

5. The nurse should plan to administer a patient's cyclophosphamide (Cytoxan) therapy in the early morning:

   a. in order to monitor the patient during waking hours.

   b. to assure increase distribution of the drug with activity.

   c. to assure giving several meals after its administration.

   *d. to prevent its accumulation in the bladder at night.

   Reference: p. 760

6. An oncologist prescribes fluorouracil (5-FU) 12 mg/kg IV once daily for 4 days as palliative treatment for a patient with carcinoma of the colon. Which response by the nurse to the patient's inquiry about how the drug works is correct?

   * a. "It is an antimetabolite that interferes with DNA synthesis."

   b. "It is an alkylating agent that causes cross-linking of DNA."

   c. "It is a natural product that blocks the production of enzymes."

   d. "It is a hormonal agent that blocks tumor cell receptor sites."

   Reference: p. 760

7. In the patient receiving fluorouracil (5-FU), nursing assessment would include monitoring the patient for the commonly occurring side effect of:

   a. petit-mal seizures.

   b. hemorrhagic cystitis.

   *c. gastritis.

   d. muscle pain.

   Reference: p. 760

8. A condition that would indicate the need for the cautious use of fluorouracil (5-FU) is:

   a. an elevated fasting blood sugar.

   *b. hyperuricemia.

   c. cardiac arrhythmia.

d. decreased forced expiratory volume.

Reference: p. 760

9. Health teaching for patients taking fluorouracil therapy would include instructions to:

   *a. report dark, tarry stools.

   b. maintain a high protein diet.

   c. consume foods high in fiber.

   d. restrict fluid intake.

   Reference: p. 763

10. A patient is being treated for testicular cancer with bleomycin therapy. A dose-related complication seen with cumulative doses of bleomycin (Blenoxane) of greater than 400 units for which the nurse should assess the patient is:

    a. neurotoxicity.

    *b. pulmonary fibrosis.

    c. renal suppression.

    d. cardiac failure.

    Reference: p. 765

11. A unique action of plicamycin (Mithracin) making it particularly useful in the treatment of some types of cancer is that it has the effect of:

    *a. lowering the serum calcium.

    b. decreasing potassium excretion.

    c. controlling hyperuricemia.

    d. preventing cystitis.

    Reference: p. 768

Vivian Houston, a patient with ovarian carcinoma, is admitted to the Oncology Clinical Unit for combination therapy with IV doxorubicin (Andriamycin-RDF) and cisplatin Reference: Reference latinol).

12. Nursing interventions for the patient receiving cisplatin latinol therapy, particularly if given concurrently with loop diuretics, would include monitoring for:

    a. hypoglycemia.

    *b. ototoxicity.

    c. hematuria.

    d. rales and wheezes.

    Reference: p. 760

13. The nurse should closely monitor the patient receiving IV doxorubicin (Adriamycin-RDF) for:

    a. thrombophlebitis of the vein into which it is being infused.

    *b. extravasation of the drug at the site of IV cannualization.

    c. pulmonary embolism secondary to venous thrombosis.

d. tetany secondary to decreased ionized serum calcium.

Reference: p. 767

14. Prior to administering the prescribed doxorubicin (Adriamycin-RDF), the nurse reviews the patient's medication history. A drug taken concurrently with doxorubicin that may prolong its half-life, thereby necessitating a reduction in the recommended dosage is:

    a. acetaminophen (Tylenol)

    b. warfarin sodium (Coumadin)

    c. vitamin B$_{12}$

    *d. streptozocin (Zanosar).

    Reference: p. 770

15. With doxorubicin (Adriamycin-RDF) administration it is essential that the nurse closely monitor the patient's:

    a. serum BUN and creatinine levels.

    b. serum uric acid levels.

    *c. electrocardiogram.

    d. serum calcium levels.

    Reference: p. 770

16. The nurse caring for the patient who is receiving doxorubicin (Adriamycin-RDF) should frequently assess them for:

    *a. dyspnea, tachycardia.

    b. paralytic ileus, constipation.

    c. erythema, hyperpigmentation.

    d. mental confusion, drowsiness.

    Reference: p. 771

17. The nurse should inform the patient who is receiving doxorubicin (Adriamycin-RDF) that a common side effect that is experienced is:

    a. diplopia for 2 to 3 days following therapy.

    b. muscle weakness for 24 hours after therapy.

    *c. red urine for 2 to 4 days after drug administration.

    d. transient water retention for 3 to 4 days.

    Reference: p. 771

Terrance Moore, a 35 year old sculptor, is admitted to the Oncology Clinical Unit for treatment of disseminated Hodgkin's lymphoma (stage IIB). He is being treated with combination chemotherapy regimen known as *MOPP* — mechlorethamine (Nitrogen Mustard), vincristine (Oncovin), procarbazine (Matulane), and prednisone.

18. The rationale for the choice of combination chemotherapy regimens for the treatment of lymphomas include all of the following *except*:

    a. they delay the emergence of resistance in tumor cells.

b. cell growth is interrupted at multiple points in the cell cycle.

*c. drugs mutually cancel the side effects of all the others given.

d. they produce longer periods of remission than with a single agent.

Reference: pgs. 791—793

19. Nursing interventions for the patient receiving vincristine (Oncovin) therapy should include assessment of:

*a. of deep tendon reflexes.

b. of level of consciousness.

c. of respiratory function.

d. for anaphylactic-like reactions.

Reference: p. 769

20. The nurse would correctly plan to administer the prescribed vincristine (Oncovin):

a. intramuscularly.

b. orally.

*c. intravenously.

d. intrathecally.

Reference: p. 769

21. The antitumor effects of the prednisone in the MOP Pregimen used in the treatment of Hodgkin's lymphoma is based on:

a. suppression of normal pituitary ACTH production.

b. inhibiting transport of growth hormone into tumor cells.

*c. binding to the corticosteriod receptors on the tumor cells.

d. competition with sex hormones for tumor cell binding sites.

Reference: p. 771

22. Because of the inclusion of procarbazine (Matulane) in a *MOPP* drug regimen for Hodgkin's lymphoma, the nurse should caution the patient against:

*a. ethanol ingestion in any form.

b. intake of foods high in calcium.

c. intake of potassium rich foods.

d. ingestion of foods high in sodium.

Reference: p. 778

23. Nursing assessment of the patient on a *MOPP* drug regimen for Hodgkin's lymphoma would include close monitoring of:

a. liver function tests.

b. serum amylase and lipase.

c. serum electrolyte levels.

*d. WBC, RBC, and thrombocyte counts.

Reference: p. 778

24. Because of a common side effect occurring with the *MOPP* treatment regimen for Hodgkin's lymphoma, health teaching would include instructing the patient to promptly report:

a. weakness.

b. fatigue.

*c. fever.

d. depression.

Reference: p. 778

25. Patients with neoplastic disease who experience the greatest benefit from hormone therapy are those:

a. who's tumors are lacking in estrogen receptors.

*b. who have receptor-containing tumors.

c. not benefiting from other antineoplastic agents.

d. needing sensitization to the effects of other agents.

Reference: p. 772

26. Rose Mancasola, a 66 year old female being treated with tamoxifen (Nolvadex) for breast carcinoma asks the nurse to explain it's mechanism of action. The nurse's answer is based on the knowledge that this hormone-altering antineoplastic agent acts by:

a. altering the effects of somatotropic hormone.

b. binding progesterone as it is produced.

c. neutralizing testosterone from the adrenal gland.

*d. being specifically antagonistic to estrogen.

Reference: p. 772

27. In addition to the RBC, WBC and differential, and thrombocyte counts, assessment of the patient being treated with tamoxifen (Nolvadex) includes monitoring laboratory values for:

a. serum magnesium levels.

*b. serum calcium levels.

c. serum albumin levels.

d. alkaline phosphate levels.

Reference: p. 772

28. Because of a significant adverse reaction associated with its use, which of the following nursing diagnoses would apply to the patient on long-term tamoxifen (Nolvadex) therapy?

a. High risk for impaired gas exchange.

b. High risk for injury secondary to muscle weakness.

*c. High risk for sensory/perceptual alteration (visual).

d. High risk for fluid volume excess.

Reference: p. 775

NOTES

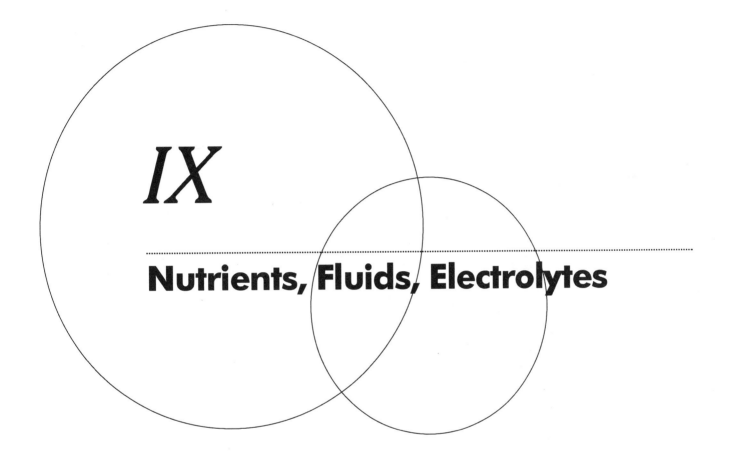

IX

Nutrients, Fluids, Electrolytes

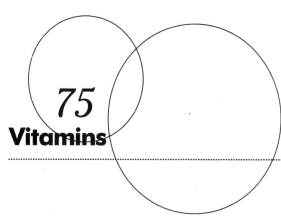

75
Vitamins

1. If a deficiency of a vitamin can be proven, the clinical approach for treatment is to:

   *a. provide selective replacement of the lacking vitamins based on symptoms.

   b. correct the deficiency with multivitamin therapy.

   c. replacement of the lacking vitamins based on lab work.

   d. replacement of vitamins in "megadose" amounts.

   Reference: p. 797

2. Vitamin deficiency states can result from all *except*:

   a. stress.

   b. hyperthyroidism.

   c. carcinoma.

   *d. american dietary habits.

   Reference: p. 797

4. The symptoms of premenstrual syndrome (PMS) can be relieved by:

   a. niacin.

   b. pantothenic acid.

   c. cyanocobalamin.

   *d. pyridoxine.

   Reference: p. 798

5. A deficiency in thiamine (vitamin B-1) results in:

   a. pellagra.

   *b. beriberi

   c. scurvy.

   d. rickets.

   Reference: p. 797

6. One of your clients is to receive IV thiamine therapy for treatment of thiamine deficiency secondary to alcoholism. Before you start the IV, your appropriate nursing action is to:

   a. assess for skin lesions.

   b. mix in 10cc of Normal Saline and prepare to give as an IV push.

   *c. perform an intradermal sensitivity test.

   d. mix with 100cc NaCl and prepare to give as a piggyback.

   Reference: p. 800

7. Adverse reactions to thiamine include:

   a. tachycardia.

   b. hypotension.

   c. flushing of the skin.

   *d. dyspnea.

   Reference: p. 800

8. Riboflavin is found in:

   *a. green vegetables.

   b. pork.

   c. yellow vegetables.

   d. fruit.

   Reference: p. 798

9. When mixed together in solution, riboflavin interacts with:

   a. ascorbic Acid.

   b. penicillin.

   *c. tetracycline.

   d. digitalis.

   Reference: p. 801

10. Advise your client taking large doses of niacin to expect:

    a. immediate cessation of deficiency symptoms.

    *b. flushing, itching of the skin.

    c. feelings of lethargy.

    d. transient visual diplopia.

    Reference: p. 802

11. Niacin is useful in the treatment of:

    a. dermatitis.

    b. acne.

*c. hyperlipidemia.

d. optic neuritis.

Reference: p. 802

12. You note that your patient is taking an oral contraceptive. You are aware that the requirement of which vitamin is increased with the use of oral contraceptives?

a. Cyanocobalamin (vitamin B-12).

b. Folic acid (vitamin B-9).

c. Thiamine (vitamin B-1).

*d. Pyridoxine (vitamin B-6).

Reference: p. 803

13. Overdosage of vitamin A is associated with the adverse reactions of:

a. tachycardia, dyspnea.

b. photophobia, constipation.

c. edema, decreased circulation.

*d. jaundice, dry skin.

Reference: p. 806

14. Foods high in vitamin D include:

a. red meat.

b. citrus fruit.

*c. egg yolk.

d. yellow vegetables.

Reference: p. 798

15. One of your patients is taking a vitamin D preparation, but is also taking Digitalis. Because of the interaction between Digitalis and vitamin D, you realize that your patient is at risk for:

a. decreased vitamin D absorption necessitating increased dosages.

b. increased risk of overdosage of vitamin D due to increased absorption.

c. increased deficiency of other fat soluble vitamins.

*d. increased likelihood of cardiac arrhythmias.

Reference: p. 808

16. Your patient is recovering from a CVA and is taking Coumadin to decrease his risk of deep vein thromboses. He has been reading in the popular press about the virtues of vitamin E in the prevention of heart disease and asks you about the advisability of taking regular doses of this vitamin while he is taking coumadin. You inform him that:

a. vitamin E deficiency is common as our diet does not supply adequate amounts.

b. vitamin E may reduce the effectiveness of coumadin.

*c. vitamin E may increase his risk of bleeding while he is on coumadin therapy.

d. vitamin E has no effect on anticoagulant therapy.

Reference: p. 809

17. The vitamin whose action enables the liver to produce clotting factors is:

a. vitamin E.

*b. vitamin K.

c. vitamin C.

d. vitamin A.

Reference: p. 809

18. All of those listed may need vitamin supplementation *except:*

a. Mrs. C., who is recovering from an infection of surgical wound.

b. Eighty-two year old Mr. S., who lives in a board and care facility.

c. Mr. D., who smokes 1 1/2 packs a day.

*d. Ms. U., who abstains from eating meat three times per week.

Reference: p. 799

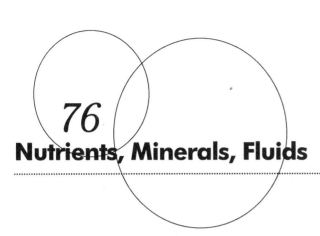

76
Nutrients, Minerals, Fluids

1. Mr. K. presents in the emergency room with the symptoms of lethargy, muscle cramping and irregular heartbeats. Electrolyte studies show that he is in a state of hypokalemia. What other electrolyte is also low when potassium is depleted?

   a. calcium.

   b. sodium.

   c. magnesium.

   *d. chloride.

   Reference: p. 812

2. As Mr. K. is hypokalemic, you review his history and medications with him. What is a common cause of hypokalemia?

   a. excessive sodium loss.

   *b. diuretic use.

   c. excessive water intake.

   d. renal failure.

   Reference: p. 812

3. Mr. K.'s serum potassium level 2.0. His physician prescribes intravenous potassium to correct his hypokalemia. Which order would you question?

   *a. 2 mEq of Potassium Chloride IV bolus.

   b. potassium chloride 5 mEq/hour IV for 24 hours.

   c. potassium chloride 10 mEq/ hour IV for 20 hours.

   d. potassium chloride 15 mEq/hour IV for 12 hours.

   Reference: p. 817

4. As you take Mr. K.'s history prior beginning his medication for hypokalemia, what would alert you that potassium is contraindicated for him?

   a. advanced cardiac disease.

   b. severe hepatic disfunction.

   *c. severe renal impairment.

   d. bone marrow depression.

   Reference: p. 815

5. As Mr. K.'s IV potassium is begun, you monitor his response to the therapy. What is a possible adverse reaction to potassium?

   a. blood dyscrasia.

   *b. cardiac arrhythmias.

   c. renal shutdown.

   d. anaphylactic shock.

   Reference: p. 817

6. After IV therapy, Mr. K. is placed on maintenance therapy with an oral potassium preparation. Your patient teaching includes the statement:

   a. "Potassium should be taken between meals."

   b. "Potassium should be taken on an empty stomach."

   c. "Salt substitutes should be used when you are taking potassium supplements."

   *d. "Swallow the pills with a whole glass of water."

   Reference: p. 818

7. Uses for choline include symptom relief of:

   a. hyperlipidemia.

   *b. CNS disorders.

   c. PMS.

   d. circulatory disorders.

   Reference: p. 814

8. Total parenteral nutrition (TPN) is indicated under these conditions:

   *a. severe burns.

   b. electrolyte imbalance.

   c. viral diarrhea.

   d. hyperthermia.

   Reference: p. 819

9. TPN is contraindicated for all of these patients except:

   a. Mr. C., who is experiencing dyspnea from pulmonary edema and fluid overload.

   b. Mr. A., who is suffering from septicemia which has precipitated an adrenal crisis.

   c. Mrs. R., who has become oliguric from acute renal failure.

*d. Mrs. Y., who is dehydrated, not taking food well, and has become hypokalemic.

Reference: p. 820

10. Appropriate nursing actions during TPN include:

a. frequent blood pressure and pulse checks.

b. adding intravenous medications to the solution.

c. withdrawing blood samples from the indwelling catheter.

*d. monitoring blood sugar levels frequently.

Reference: p. 821

11. An example of an isotonic dextrose solution is:

a. D-2 1/2-W.

*b. D-5-W.

c. D-10-W.

d. D-20-W.

Reference: p. 821

12. An example of an isotonic sodium solution is one with a concentration of:

a. 0.45%.

*b. 0.9%

c. 3%

d. 5%

Reference: p. 817

13. The IV sodium solution concentration used most frequently for fluid and sodium replacement is:

a. 0.45%

*b. 0.9%.

c. 3%

d. 5%

Reference: p. 817

14. Laboratory studies that must be monitored during infusion of fat emulsions include:

a. LDH, CPK.

b. blood glucose levels.

c. renal function tests.

*d. liver function, platelet counts.

Reference: p. 824

15. When administering fat emulsions with dextrose and amino acid solutions, appropriate nursing actions include:

*a. using a Y connector, hang the lipid infusion line higher than the dextrose-amino acid line.

b. if the solution cannot be used immediately, freeze the solution at -42°C.

c. infuse the two together, using a volume control set.

d. infuse the two together through a fine mesh filter.

Reference: p. 824

16. Your patient's TPN solution has arrived from the pharmacy and you notice that the emulsions appear to have separated out of the solution. Your action is to:

a. shake the solution.

b. gently roll the bag to mix.

c. warm the mixture.

*d. discard the emulsion.

Reference: p. 824

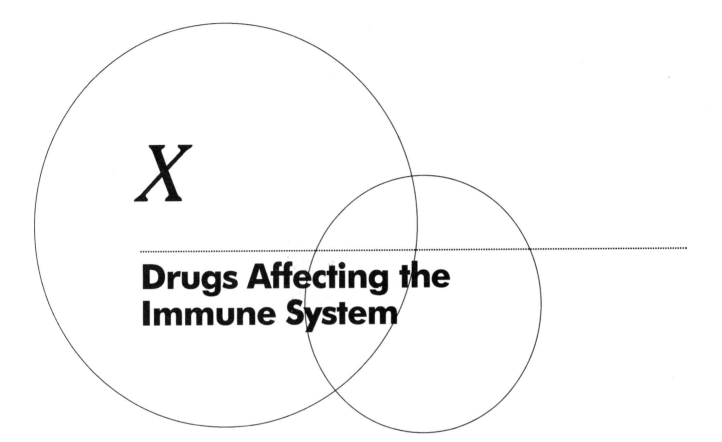

X

Drugs Affecting the Immune System

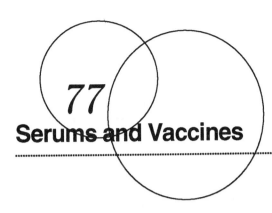

77
Serums and Vaccines

1. An example of an agent used for active immunity is:

    a. diphtheria antitoxin.

    b. immune globulins.

    c. antirabies serum.

    *d. hepatitis B vaccine.

    Reference: p. 829

2. Antitoxins and antivenins are prepared by:

    *a. immunizing an animal against a disease and removing and purifying the serum.

    b. formulating a suspension of killed microorganisms that are capable of stimulating antibody production.

    c. formulating a suspension of inactivated microorganisms that are capable of stimulating antibody production.

    d. preparing globulins possessing antibodies against various diseases.

    Reference: pgs. 829—835

3. Your client has presented herself at your clinic for a measles vaccination. You give her information about the vaccine that includes the statement:

    *a. "This vaccine contains the virus that causes measles, but they have been changed so that they no longer cause the disease."

    b. "This is a vaccine made from preformed antibodies from a human or animal source."

    c. "You are less likely to have an allergic reaction to this vaccination. "

    d. "Before we can give this vaccine to you, we will have to perform a skin test to be sure that you are not sensitive to it."

    Reference: p. 834

4. Live virus vaccines should *not* be given to persons who are:

    a. elderly.

    b. suffering with cold symptoms.

    *c. ill with leukemia.

    d. diagnosed with myasthenia gravis.

    Reference: p. 830

5. BCG is *contraindicated* in:

    a. the presence of symptoms of malaise and fever.

    *b. tuberculin-positive patients.

    c. patients with hepatitis.

    d. patients receiving other vaccinations concurrently.

    Reference: p. 832

6. Which of these patients should not receive the influenza vaccine?

    a. Mrs. S, who is 72 years old.

    *b. Mr. B., who is wheezing and febrile.

    c. Mr. H., who suffers from mild congestive heart failure.

    d. Mrs. D., who suffers from chronic renal failure.

    Reference: p. 833

7. The pneumococcal vaccine is not recommended for:

    a. debilitated persons.

    b. those with frequent otitis media.

    *c. those under two years of age.

    d. the elderly population.

    Reference: p. 832

8. Tetanus toxoid should not be given when a client is taking:

    *a. vincristine.

    b. theophylline.

    c. epinephrine.

    d. cefaclor.

    Reference: p. 831

9. Immunity to mumps is conferred for how long after vaccination?

    a. 5 years.

    *b. 10 years.

    c. 20 years.

    d. for life.

Reference: p. 884

10. The advantages in the use of human immune globulins rather than serums from animal sources include:

    a. longer lasting immunity.

    b. lower cost for administration.

    c. they are more readily available.

    *d. fewer hypersensitive reactions.

Reference: p. 831

11. Administration of Crotalidae Antivenin to treat snakebite is most effective if it is given by:

    a. injecting the area around the bite.

    *b. intravenous infusion.

    c. a single IM injection.

    d. a series of IM injections.

Reference: p. 835

12. Your patient has had immune globulin 1 g IV, prescribed in order to provide a rapid increase in IgG antibody levels. Your appropriate nursing action during the infusion is to:

    a. monitor the patient's temperature frequently.

    b. check for bleeding frequently.

    *c. monitor the blood pressure carefully.

    d. check for urticaria frequently.

Reference: p. 836

13. During an infusion of immune globulin, it is prudent for the nurse to keep on hand:

    a. probenecid.

    b. theophylline.

    c. benadryl.

    *d. epinephrine.

Reference: p. 936

14. After exposure to rabies, the best protection is conferred by:

    a. rabies vaccine, human diploid cultures.

    b. rabies immune globulin.

    c. antirabies serum, equine.

    *d. several doses of vaccine and rabies immune globulin.

Reference: p. 837

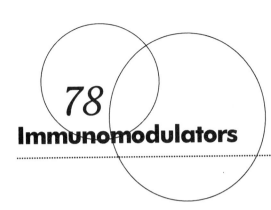

78
Immunomodulators

1. Acquired (adaptive) immunity differs from natural (innate) immunity because it is:

   a. the first line of defense.

   b. able to defend the body against a wide array of bacteria.

   c. involved in the inflammatory response.

   *d. a specific immune response.

   Reference: p. 839

2. Cells specific to the adaptive immune response are called:

   a. neutrophils

   b. monocytes.

   *c. lymphocytes.

   d. eosinophils.

   Reference: p. 839

3. The cells that do not function as subsets of T lymphocytes are:

   a. helper/inducer cells.

   *b. plasma cells.

   c. cytotoxic (killer) cells.

   d. supressor cells.

   Reference: p. 839

4. The role of suppressor T Cells in the immune response includes:

   a. amplification of B cell activity.

   b. stimulation of proliferation of activated T 8 cells.

   c. destruction of cell membranes.

   *d. inhibition of B cell responses to antigens.

   Reference: p. 840

5. The specific immunoglobulin which binds to mast cells and is involved in allergic (immediate) hypersensitivity states is:

   a. IgA

   b. IgD

   c. IgB

   *d. IgE

   Reference: p. 841

6. Of the following, the statement which does not apply to IgG (immunoglobulin G) is:

   a. IgG is the major circulatory antibody in the blood.

   *b. IgG is involved in the "primary response" to antigens.

   c. IgG is capable of crossing the placenta.

   d. IgG is secreted during the secondary response to antigens.

   Reference: p. 840

7. Principal indications for immunomodulator therapy consist of all *except*:

   a. prevention of organ transplantation rejection.

   b. treatment of autoimmune disease.

   c. correction of primary immunodeficiency disorders.

   *d. adjunct treatment for patients receiving antiplatelet therapy.

   Reference: p. 842

8. Sargramostim (Leukine) is useful for:

   *a. Enhancing bone marrow recovery after radiation.

   b. Preventing the rejection of transplanted tissues.

   c. Prolonging graft survival.

   d. Treatment of macrocytic anemia.

   Reference: p. 843

9. In addition to use as an immunosuppressive agent, azathioprine (Imuran) is useful for:

   a. enhancement of the immune system by stimulation of B-cell growth.

   *b. treating severe rheumatoid arthritis.

   c. blocking the action of interleukin-1.

   d. treating patients receiving antiplatelet therapy.

   Reference: p. 843

10. What nursing assessments are important during therapy with interferon beta-1 b (Betaseron)?

   a. Cardiac and pulmonary auscultation for arrhythmias and congestion.

   b. Careful intake and output, monitor labs for rising nitrogen levels.

   *c. Assessment for fever, sore throat, complaints of fatigue.

   d. Observe skin color, palpate abdomen for upper right quadrant tenderness.

Reference: p. 848

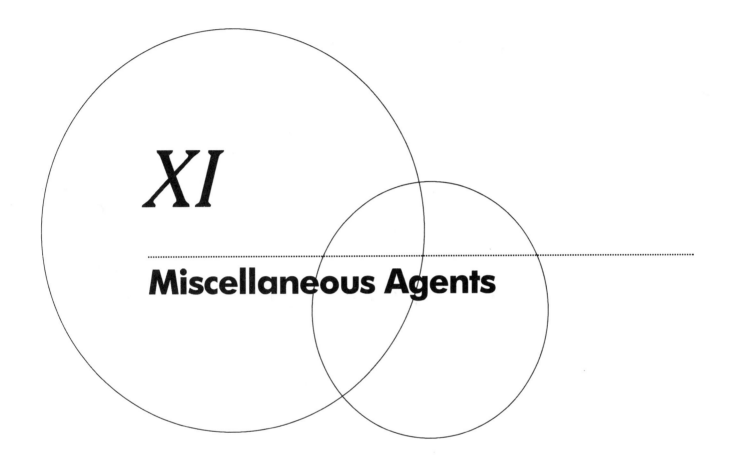

XI

Miscellaneous Agents

79
Dermatologic Agents

1. The patient being treated for acne vulgaris asks the nurse the action of tretinoin (Retin-A) on the acne lesions. The nurse correctly responds:

   *a. "It promotes cell turnover and facilitates desquamation."

   b. "It facilitates keratin synthesis and stops desquamation."

   c. "It inhibits sebaceous gland differentiation."

   d. "It decreases the thickness of the lesions and drys them."

   Reference: p. 853

2. Tara Martini, 17 years old, is being treated by a dermatologist for acne vulgaris who prescribes tretinoin (Retin-A) to be applied topically to the affected areas. The nurse should instruct the patient to:

   a. avoid washing the skin with drying soaps.

   *b. limit exposure to sunlamps and sunlight.

   c. decrease intake of caffeine containing foods.

   d. discontinue the drug if a stinging feeling occurs.

   Reference: p. 853

3. The nurse should instruct the patient being treated for acne with tretinoin (Retin-A) that an expected effect associated with its use is:

   a. edematous blisters of the skin.

   b. temporary depigmentation.

   c. oily skin initially; dryness later.

   *d. dryness and peeling of the skin.

   Reference: p. 853

4. Patient instructions in the use of tretinoin (Retin-A) ointment for the treatment of acne lesions should include advising the patient to:

   a. use alcohol to clean the lesions prior to application.

   *b. avoid contact with mucous membranes as the eyes and mouth.

   c. expect results with in 10 days to 2 weeks.

   d. using gloves, apply a thick layer 4 times a day.

   Reference: p. 854

5. Health teaching for the patient taking isotretinoin (Accutane) for treatment of acne should include instructions to:

   *a. avoid vitamin products containing vitamin A.

   b. increase caloric intake over previous levels.

   c. take the drug on an empty stomach.

   d. expose the affected area to UV light.

   Reference: p. 855

6. Which of the following laboratory tests would the nurse expect to monitor initially and weekly or biweekly in the patient taking isotretinoin (Accutane)?

   a. calcium level.

   b. total protein level.

   *c. triglyceride level.

   d. white blood count.

   Reference: p. 856

7. Health teaching for the individual taking isotretinoin (Accutane) should include informing the patient:

   a. therapy will need to continue indefinitely.

   b. to take measures to avoid constipation.

   *c. to eliminate all alcohol intake.

   d. lesions start to disappear within 24 hours.

   Reference: p. 855

8. An over-the-counter medication commonly used to treat moderate forms of acne and having antibacterial activity against Propionibacterium acne is:

   *a. benzoyl peroxide (Fostex).

   b. providone-iodine (Betadine).

   c. benzalkonium chloride (Zephiran).

   d. triclosan (Septi-Soft).

   Reference: p. 856

9. Jimmy Warren, 6 years old, is diagnosed as having impetigo. An antibacterial agent indicated in the

treatment of impetigo due to *Staphylococcus aureus* or beta-hemolytic streptococci is:

a. bacitracin.

b. polymyxin B.

c. gentamicin.

*d. mupirocin.

Reference: p. 856

10. Cassie Stuart, 27 years old, is seen by a dermatologist for severe psoriasis unresponsive to conventional forms of therapy. The patient questions the nurse about the mechanism of action of the the prescribed etretinate (Tegison). The correct response by the nurse is:

a. "It causes desquamation and blocks keratin synthesis."

b. "It inhibits sebaceous gland differentiation."

*c. "It decreases erythema and thickness of the lesions."

d. "It is antipruritic, and promotes keratoplastic activity."

Reference: p. 857

11. Health education of the patient using etretinate (Tegison) for treatment of psoriasis should emphasize:

a. it's potential for causing sterility.

*b. the drug's teratogenic potential.

c. possible associated agranulocytosis.

d. the need to avoid use of vitamin C.

Reference: p. 858

12. Henretta Lewis, 81 years old, is being treated for a pressure ulcer. The category to which the dermatologic agent that may be used topically for the purpose of debriding the wound is an:

*a. enzyme.

b. corticosteroid.

c. antipsoriatic.

d. antihistamine.

Reference: p. 859

13. The drug used for treatment of the patient who has condylomata acuminatum (genital warts) is:

a. salicylic acid (Freezone).

b. canthardin (Cantherone).

c. urea (Carmol 10).

*d. podophyllum resin (Podofin).

Reference: p. 860

14. Scottie Navarro presents at the outpatient clinic of a local HMO with complaints of intense itching and dermatologic signs indicative of scabies confined to his waist area. His physician prescribes lindane (Kwell) lotion for treatment. The nurse correctly instructs the patient to:

a. apply the lotion to the entire body; leave it for 24 hours.

b. apply the lotion to the affected area; leave it for 6 hours.

c. apply the lotion to the affected area; repeat in 6 hours.

*d. apply the lotion to the affected area; leave if for 12 hours.

Reference: p. 863

16. How many days after initial treatment of scabies with lindane (Kwell) lotion may the treatment need to be repeated?

a. 3 days.

b. 5 days.

*c. 7 days.

d. 9 days.

Reference: p. 863

17. To avoid significant percutaneous absorption of the lindane (Kwell) which may result in CNS stimulation, the patient should be instructed to avoid simultaneous use of:

a. vitamin products and foods high in Vitamin A.

*b. oil based lotions and shampoos.

c. exposure to bright sunlight.

d. warm environmental temperatures.

Reference: p. 863

80 Diagnostic Agents

1. Intradermal skin tests are used to determine an individual's sensitization to all of the following diseases *except*:

   a. tuberculosis mycobacterium.

   *b. human immunodeficiency virus.

   c. histoplasmosis fungus.

   d. coccidioidomycosis fungus.

   Reference: p. 864

2. A positive local hypersensitivity reaction to an intradermal diagnostic skin test usually consists of:

   a. a soft macular area of erythema.

   b. annular vesiculation of the area.

   *c. an area of induration and redness.

   d. a circumscribed maculopapular area.

   Reference: p. 864

3. A positive response to intradermal coccidiodin:

   a. could possibly be a false positive reaction.

   *b. indicates contact with the fungus in the past.

   c. rules out contact with coccidioidomycosis.

   d. may be an allergic response sodium chloride.

   Reference: p. 867

4. Individuals who are allergic to chicken, eggs, or feathers should not receive the intradermal diagnostic biological:

   a. coccidioidin.

   b. diphtheria.

   *c. mumps antigen.

   d. histoplasmin.

   Reference: p. 867

5. In the patient that has had previous BCG vaccination, a false- positive reaction may occur with the use of:

   a. coccidioidin.

   b. trichophyton.

   *c. tuberculin PPD.

   d. histoplasmin.

   Reference: p. 867

6. The contrast agents principally employed in radiographic diagnostic procedures are:

   *a. iodinated compounds.

   b. dyes.

   c. radiolabeled agents.

   d. special gases.

   Reference: p. 870

7. A 68 year old female with possible regional enteritis is admitted for diagnostic studies. Following the a small bowel series which requires that the patient swallow barium sulfate, nursing interventions would include:

   a. restricting fluids for 8 hours.

   *b. a plan to administer a laxative.

   c. providing a soft diet.

   d. encouraging additional rest.

   Reference: p. 874

8. A 50 year old male is admitted to the medical acute care unit with complaints of intense flank pain and hematuria and his physician schedules him for an intravenous pyelogram that will employ the use of Hypaque-M 75%. A nursing history prior to the procedure would include investigation for a possible:

   a. intake of thyroid compounds.

   b. hypersensitivity to eggs.

   c. use of OTC cough syrups.

   *d. allergy to iodine.

   Reference: p. 874

81
Miscellaneous Drug Products

1. The pediatrician caring for a neonate with patent ductus arteriosus weighing 2 kg prescribes IV prostaglandin E_1 (Alprostadil). Nursing interventions would include closely assessing the infant's:

   *a. arterial blood gases.

   b. skin around the IV site.

   c. deep tendon reflexes.

   d. level of consciousness.

   Reference: p. 871

2. The effectiveness of activated charcoal in the treatment of ingested poisons is related to:

   a. its ability to neutralize most substances.

   b. its effect of causing emesis after ingestion.

   c. its effect of increased peristalsis and elimination.

   *d. is great absorptive capacity per unit weight.

   Reference: p. 877

3. A 3 year old child ingests large quantities of his mother's candy-coated ferrous sulfate (iron) that has been prescribed for anemia. A heavy metal antidote the nurse would expect to be used in the treatment of acute iron intoxication is:

   a. edetate calcium disodium.

   *b. deferoxamine mesylate.

   c. dimercaprol-BAL.

   d. cellulose sodium phosphate.

   Reference: p. 877

4. A physician prescribes trientine (Cuprid) for a patient diagnosed with Wilson's disease. The nurse assesses the laboratory values indicative of a positive response to the drug which is exhibited by a decreased serum level of:

   a. magnesium.

   b. calcium.

   *c. copper.

   d. zinc.

   Reference: p. 877

5. Health teaching for patient taking trientine (Cuprid) includes instructions to increase the intake of:

   a. dairy products as yogurt and milk.

   *b. red meat, dark green vegetables.

   c. foods high in insoluble fiber.

   d. potassium-rich foods.

   Reference: p. 888

6. Manny Cisco, 3 years old, is diagnosed as having lead poisoning. His physician prescribe succimer (Chemet) 10 mg/kg orally. Health teaching should include instructing the patient's mother to administer the medication:

   a. 3 times a day for 2 days.

   b. 2 times a day for 5 day.

   *c. every 8 hours for 5 days.

   d. every 12 hours for 7 days.

   Reference: p. 840

7. A patient with recurrent nephrolithiasis caused by calcium oxalate renal stones is taking cellulose sodium phosphate (Calcibind). The nurse correctly explains to the patient that the mechanism of action of this drug is:

   *a. binding of calcium in the gut and excretion.

   b. augmented renal calcium excretion.

   c. decrease in calcium release from bones.

   d. increased calcium deposition in the bones.

   Reference: p. 840

8. A condition that would be a contraindication to the use of cellulose sodium phosphate (Calcibind) is:

   a. hypothyroidism

   b. diabetes mellitus

   *c. hyperparathyroidism

   d. Cushing's syndrome

   Reference: p. 879

9. For the patient taking cellulose sodium phosphate (Calcibind) planned nursing interventions would include:

   a. increased dietary intake of vitamin C-rich foods.

   *b. fluid intake to maintain a 2,000 ml/24 hour output.

   c. periodic monitoring of serum liver enzyme levels.

   d. baseline measurement of abdominal girth.

   Reference: p. 879

10. A patient with acromegaly is admitted to a acute care medical unit for pituitary irradiation. A drug that is sometimes used in addition to pituitary irradiation for treatment of acromegaly is:

    a. hemin (Panhematin).

    b. papain (Panafil).

    *c. bromocriptine (Parlodel).

    d. flavoxate (Urispas).

    Reference: p. 880

11. A physician orders capsaicin (Zostrix) cream to alleviate residual pain in a patient following the healing of herpes zoster lesions. Health education for the patient should include instructing the patient that a warm or burning sensation can occur with application if:

    *a. it is applied less than 3-4 times a day.

    b. polyester clothing is worn over it.

    c. the individual is allergic to xylocaine.

    d. applied 4 times a day every day.

    Reference: p. 880

12. A physician prescribes bladder instillations of dimethyl sulfoxide (Rimso-50) for patient with symptomatic interstitial cystitis. Patient education should include informing the patient that with administration of the drug they may experience:

    a. slight dysuria and dark reddish-brown urine.

    b. fleeting skin flushing and a sensation of warmth.

    *c. a garlic-like odor or taste appearing in a few minutes.

    d. transient gagging and a bitter taste in their mouth.

    Reference: p. 881

13. The nurse should warn the patient that after disulfiram (Antabuse) intake is discontinued a mal rouge reaction to alcohol ingestion can occur for as long as:

    a. 1 week.

    *b. 2 weeks.

    c. 4 weeks.

    d. 8 weeks.

    Reference: p. 881

14. Health teaching for the patient with alcoholism for which disulfiram (Antabuse) is prescribed should include informing the patient that:

    a. it will cure alcoholism in selected patients.

    b. it increases metabolism of alcohol.

    *c. it it acts as a deterrent to drinking.

    d. it decreases absorption of alcohol.

    Reference: p. 881

15. Nursing interventions for an elderly patient receiving fluids by hypodermoclysis to which hyluronidase (Wydase) has been added includes monitoring for:

    *a. overhydration.

    b. dysuria.

    c. hypertension.

    d. pericardial friction rub

    Reference: p. 883

16. A nursing diagnoses that applies to the patient taking flavoxate (Urispas) is:

    a. High risk for sleep pattern disturbance related to fatigue

    *b. High risk alteration in mucous membranes related to dry mouth

    c. High risk for hyperthermia related to dehydration

    d. High risk for altered bowel function: Diarrhea related to medication side-effects.

    Reference: p. 884

17. A patient diagnosed as having intermittent porphyria has an acute attack of the disease. The drug most likely to be prescribed for this disorder is:

    *a. hemin (Panhematin).

    b. sutilains (Travase).

    c. cyclosporine (Sandimmune).

    d. collagenase (Biozyme-C).

    Reference: p. 884

18. Rhandhawa Nangpali is receiving gallium nitrate (Ganite for the treatment of cancer-related hypercalcemia. The drug would be contraindicated in the patient with a:

    a. serum calcium of <9 mg/dl

    *b. serum creatinine >2.5 mg/dl

    c. serum alanine aminotrasferase level <24 U/L.

    d. serum alkaline phosphatase of <70 U/L.

    Reference: p. 884

19. A physician prescribes mesalamine (Rowasa) for a patient with chronic proctitis. Health teaching will include patient instructions to take the medication as:

    a. orally with a soft diet.

    b. a rectal suppository after defecation.

    *c. a retention enema at bedtime.

    d. as a subcutaneous injection.

    Reference: p. 885

20. The mechanism by which mesalamine (Rowasa) exerts it anti-inflammatory action on the colon is through:

    a. producing a rapid decline in T cell production.

    b. reversibly inhibiting T lymphocyte synthesis.

    c. interfering with nucleic acid and protein synthesis.

    *d. inhibiting the production of prostaglandins.

    Reference: p. 885

21. Although there are no absolute contraindications to the use ofmesalamine (Rowasa), it should be used cautiously in patients with a known allergic response to:

    a. penicillin derivatives.

    *b. sulfa drugs.

    c. antifungal agents.

    d. antiviral drugs.

    Reference: p. 885

22. A drug used for the symptomatic treatment of patients with metastatic carcinoid tumors to alleviate symptoms of severe diarrhea and flushing is:

    *a. octreotide (Sandostatin).

    b. olsalazine (Dipentum).

    c. pegademase bovine (Adagen).

    d. perfluorochemical emulsion (Fluosol).

    Reference: p. 886

23. A patient admitted to the emergency department for acute shock secondary to severe blood loss is given IV dextran, low molecular weight (Dextran 40). The effects of this drug is mediated through:

    a. arteriolar vasoconstriction with increased blood pressure.

    b. stimulation of the renin mechanism with vasoconstriction.

    *c. increased blood osmotic pressure and intravascular volume.

    d. reflex vasoconstriction from baroreceptor stimulation.

    Reference: p. 887

24. Intravenous dextran is used in patients undergoing high-risk surgical procedures as in hip-replacement operations to prevent:

    a. compromised myocardial perfusion and infarction.

    b. decreased cerebral perfusion and stroke..

    c. reduced renal perfusion and renal failure.

    *d. venous thrombosis and pulmonary embolism.

    Reference: p. 887

25. Nursing interventions for the patient receiving IV dextran include monitoring for and reporting to the patient's physician a laboratory value of:

    a. potassium 3.5 mg/dl.

    b. total serum protein 7 g/dl.

    *c. hematocrit 28 mg/dl.

    d. total calcium 8.8 mg/dl.

    Reference: p. 887

26. A patient asks the nurse why his physician has prescribed albumin, human (Albuminar). The nurse correctly responds:

    a. "It expands blood volume by lowering your blood osmotic pressure."

    b. "It provides the necessary protein needed for nutritional health."

    c. "It is much safer than whole blood and you get the same effect."

    *d. "It increases intravascular volume and raises osmotic pressure."

    Reference: p. 888

27. Plasma protein fraction (Plasmanate) should be used cautiously in the patient with:

    a. hypovolemic shock.

    *b. sodium-restrictions.

    c. hypoproteinemia.

    d. fat restrictions.

    Reference: p. 889

28. Paula Rhemquist suffers from recurrent, debilitating migraine headaches for which her physician has prescribed sumatriptan (Imitrex). Health teaching for Paula should include informing her that a common side effect of the drug is:

    a. drowsiness, sleepiness, and lethargy.

    *b. a sensation of warmth and tingling.

    c. temporary urinary retention.

    d. slight edema at the injection site.

    Reference: p. 890

29. Because of its mechanism of action, sumatriptan (Imitrex) should be avoided in patients with:

    a. conductive hearing loss.

    b. muscular weakness.

c. hypotension.

*d. ischemic heart disease.

Reference: p. 891

30. Because Leo Lehnman does not respond to more conservative therapy for severe cystinuria, his physician prescribes tiopronin (Thiola). A critical nursing intervention for the patient who is taking tiopronin is monitoring of the patient for:

*a. a high volume urine output with a high pH.

b. intake of foods and fluids to acidify the urine.

c. a high volume urine output with a low pH.

d. presence of blood in the urine.

Reference: p. 892

NOTES

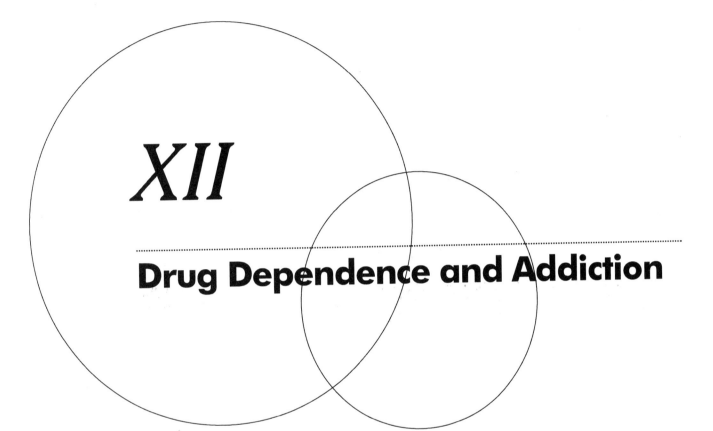

XII

Drug Dependence and Addiction

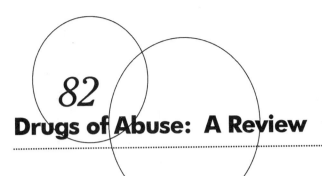

82
Drugs of Abuse: A Review

1. Broadly defined, the term "drug abuse" refers to the use of any drug that:

   a. is not prescribed and used for the intended purpose.

   b. produces bizarre behavior in a person.

   *c. deviates from the accepted sociological norm.

   d. results in psychological dependence.

   Reference: p. 897

2. Jermiah Annandale regularly takes cocaine by IV injection. His overwhelming need to experience the pleasurable sensations associated with cocaine use is descriptive of:

   a. tolerance.

   *b. psychological dependence.

   c. physical dependence.

   d. habit.

   Reference: p. 897

3. An altered physiological state resulting from prolonged drug use and accompanied by severe withdrawal reactions if the user discontinues taking it is termed:

   a. habit.

   *b. physical dependence.

   c. psychological dependence.

   d. tolerance.

   Reference: p. 897

4. Drug related fatalities most frequently occur as a result of the use of alcohol in combination with:

   a. amphetamines.

   b. marijuana.

   c. mescaline.

   *d. barbiturates.

   Reference: p. 898

5. Impaired motor coordination, concentration, and memory occur in the individual with a blood alcohol level of:

   a. 25 mg/dl.

   b. 50 mg/dl.

   *c. 100 mg/dl.

   d. 300 mg/dl.

   Reference: p. 898

6. A drug used to alleviate life threatening symptoms, as convulsions, that may occur secondary to withdrawal from chronic barbiturate dependence is:

   * a. phenobarbital.

   b. morphine sulfate.

   c. methadone.

   d. naltrexone.

   Reference: p. 898

7. Yawning, perspiration, lacrimation, sneezing, and restlessness are the initial signs of withdrawal from:

   a. psychotomimetics.

   *b. narcotics.

   c. amphetamines.

   d. alcohol.

   Reference: p. 899

8. Hadley Horas, who is addicted to Dilaudid, has entered a drug rehabilitation program in his local neighborhood. The drug he is most likely to receive to suppress withdrawal symptoms, thereby increasing the probability that he will remain drug free is:

   a. naltrexone.

   b. diazepam.

   c. lorazepam.

   *d. methadone.

   Reference: p. 900

9. A therapeutic use of delta-9-tetrahydrocannabinol (THC), the major psychoactive chemical compound found in marijuana, is:

   *a. to control of nausea and vomiting associated with cancer chemotherapy.

b. to improve the mood of patients suffering from AIDS and other chronic diseases.

c. to control the compulsive desire for a "fix" in patients withdrawing from drugs.

d. to augment the effects of analgesics to reduce the amount for pain control.

Reference: p. 901

10. Paul Neitz is a chronic user of powdered cocaine which he "snorts" by inhaling it through his nasal passages. Respiratory effects of his drug abuse for which the nurse would assess Paul include all of the following *except*:

a. rhinorrhea.

b. rhinitis.

c. perforated nasal septum.

*d. pleural effusion.

Reference: p. 902